Handbook of Emergency Anaesthes

D1761438

This book is dedicated to my mother and father

Handbook of Emergency Anaesthesia

Anne J. Sutcliffe, BSc, MB ChB, FFA RCS

Consultant Anaesthetist, Birmingham Accident Hospital

Butterworths
London Boston Durban Singapore Sydney Toronto Wellington

First published 1983

© Butterworth & Co (Publishers) Ltd 1983

British Library Cataloguing in Publication Data

Sutcliffe, Anne J.
   Handbook of emergency anaesthesia.
   1. Anaesthesia–Handbooks, manuals, etc.
   2. Emergency medical services
   I. Title
   617′.96   RF52

   ISBN 0–407–00216–2

Typeset by Scribe Design, Gillingham, Kent
Printed and bound by Butler & Tanner Ltd, London & Frome

Preface

This handbook has been written for junior anaesthetic staff. It is easily carried in the pocket of a white coat. In a true emergency where there is no time to obtain help or advice, it will be particularly useful. In less urgent situations, it should be used as an *aide-mémoire* and should *not* be regarded as a substitute for the assistance of senior colleagues.

The information contained in this book relates only to adult anaesthesia and is brief and dogmatic. The 'Further reading' lists the principal sources of this information, as a detailed list of references proved impossible to compile. Each section consists of an amalgamation of suggestions from several sources which I have attempted to collate in a form which my own experience suggests will be helpful.

To make best use of this book, the anaesthetist should familiarize himself with its layout. The techniques it describes should be practised during routine lists. New techniques are not easily learnt in the heat of an emergency. Having read the book, it will be obvious that Chapters 4 and 5 contain a limited number of drugs and techniques. These are sufficient to enable the anaesthetist to provide a safe and satisfactory emergency service. It does not, however, preclude him from using other techniques to achieve the same result.

By the time decisions about postoperative management have to be made, the emergency nature of the situation will be over. Detailed suggestions for postoperative care are, therefore, not included in this book.

A.J.S.

Acknowledgements

I would like to thank the following people to whom I owe a great debt:

My husband, Dr George R. Harrison, who read the manuscript and gave much helpful advice and criticism.

The editorial staff of Butterworths, without whose encouragement and help I would never have completed this book.

Mrs Jennifer Vahid-Ramezani, who spent many hours typing the manuscript.

My colleagues in the West Midlands, who have given helpful advice and encouragement.

Contents

Introduction

Patients who present for emergency surgery are nearly always less well prepared than those who appear on routine lists. Emergency anaesthesia and surgery are, therefore, more hazardous. The anaesthetist should remember the adage 'first, do no harm'. It is a mistake to allow the surgeon to rush the patient to theatre without adequate investigation and preparation. Always make an effort to see the patient before he is brought to theatre. The anaesthetist often has more medical knowledge than the surgeon and may diagnose significant disease which has been missed in the surgical assessment. Doctors from other specialties may give invaluable assistance in the diagnosis and management of non-surgical problems prior to the induction of anaesthesia. The final decision about the patient's fitness for anaesthesia should always be made by the person responsible for administering the anaesthetic. If in doubt, consult a senior anaesthetic colleague—it is a sign of strength, not failure, to recognize one's own inadequacies. If a senior colleague agrees to take over the case, the junior anaesthetist should continue to play an active part; valuable experience will be gained which may be helpful in the future.

Preoperative preparation

The sections on history and examination give a list of features which may affect the conduct of anaesthesia. An explanation should be sought for abnormal findings. If necessary, doctors from other specialties should be consulted. Chapter 9 outlines associated difficulties and suggests suitable anaesthetic techniques for the conditions mentioned.

Fitness for anaesthesia

To assess the patient's fitness for anaesthesia, answer the following questions.

Q1. Will the proposed operation improve the patient's life-expectancy?

Yes: see Q3.

No: see Q2.

Q2. Will the consequences of not operating as a matter of urgency cause unacceptable morbidity?

Yes: see Q3.

No: the patient should be regarded as a routine case and operation delayed until he meets normal criteria of fitness for anaesthesia.

Q3. How urgent is the operation?

Very urgent: prepare to proceed, and call for assistance if problems beyond your competence are likely to occur.

Less urgent: see Q4.

Non-urgent: the patient should be treated as a routine case.

Q4. Are there clinical features of the patient's condition which may represent an anaesthetic hazard?

Yes: see Q5.

No: prepare to proceed.

Q5. Are there any short-term measures to reduce this hazard?
   Yes: decide what measures you consider necessary and estimate the time necessary to carry them out.
   No: decide whether you are capable of anaesthetizing the patient.

In essence these questions ask, 'Should I give an anaesthetic to *this* patient for *this* operation in the *present* circumstances?'.

Having made his own decisions, the anaesthetist should discuss them with the surgeon. A joint decision on the following points should be made:

(1) The time of the operation.
(2) Preoperative treatment required and who is to administer it. If you can spare the time, it is best to do it yourself.

If there is any doubt or disagreement, senior colleagues should be consulted.

History

Presenting complaint

Make your own diagnosis, remembering that pneumonia, myocardial infarction and diabetes mellitus may present as abdominal pain. Note the differential diagnosis. Choose a technique which can be modified according to the operative findings.

Past medical history

(1) Ask specifically about rheumatic fever, hepatitis and diabetes mellitus.
(2) Excessive bleeding after tonsillectomy or dental extraction may indicate a bleeding diathesis.
(3) Ask about other current or past illnesses, particularly those requiring admission to hospital.
(4) Note any problems relating to previous anaesthetics; e.g. vomiting, chest infection, postoperative ventilation or care in an intensive therapy unit, deep vein thrombosis, pulmonary embolism, jaundice, difficult intubation. Consider the causes and the measures to prevent recurrence.

Recent medical history

Many drugs interact with anaesthetic agents—see Appendix 1.

Allergies

A patient may be allergic to rubber, iodine or adhesive strapping as well as to drugs.

Family history

Malignant hyperpyrexia and porphyria cause anaesthetic deaths. Postoperative ventilation may be necessary due to plasma cholinesterase deficiency.

Social history

(1) Cigarettes: beware of a stormy induction, postoperative chest infection, chronic bronchitis and ischaemic heart disease.
(2) Alcohol: acute intoxication causes delayed stomach emptying and a reduced requirement for induction agents. Chronic intake is associated with addiction and cirrhosis.
(3) Location of relatives/friends. After a brief general anaesthetic or a local anaesthetic, a relative or friend must be available to accompany the patient home and nurse him for the next 12–24 hours.

Direct questions

General

(1) Age.
(2) Dentition.
(3) Time of last food and drink.

Cardiovascular system

(1) *Angina:* causes include hypertension, aortic stenosis, thyrotoxicosis, anaemia and ischaemic heart disease. Angina of long duration may be due to myocardial infarction.
(2) *Palpitations:* causes include anxiety and dysrhythmias.
(3) *Orthopnoea and paroxysmal nocturnal dyspnoea:* causes include lung disease and left ventricular failure. The patient may not be able to lie flat for an operation under local anaesthesia.

(4) *Exercise tolerance:* this is often inversely proportional to the severity of heart or lung disease.

Respiratory system

(1) *Dyspnoea:* causes include many lung diseases and left ventricular failure. The patient may be unable to lie flat for an operation under local anaesthesia.
(2) *Productive cough:* beware of laryngeal spasm and coughing at induction.
(3) *Non-productive cough:* causes include early left ventricular failure, tuberculosis, laryngeal nerve palsy, distortion of trachea or bronchi, and bronchial irritability. Make the diagnosis if possible, and avoid irritant gases and drugs which cause bronchospasm.
(4) *Sputum:* pink and frothy sputum is caused by left ventricular failure. Purulent sputum indicates infection. Consider preoperative postural drainage and physiotherapy. If the sputum is mucoid, consider preoperative physiotherapy and use a technique which allows early resumption of coughing.

Gastrointestinal system

(1) *Weight loss:* serum proteins may be low, causing altered drug binding.
(2) *Nausea and vomiting:* may occur at induction. Consider passing a nasogastric tube for obstructive lesions or giving an anti-emetic.
(3) *Heartburn:* caused by a hiatus hernia. There is an increased risk of regurgitation at induction.

Genitourinary system

(1) *Poor urine output:* caused by hypovolaemia, dehydration or imminent renal failure.
(2) *Menorrhagia:* causes anaemia.

Nervous system

(1) *Dizziness:* causes include dysrhythmias, postural hypotension and cerebrovascular insufficiency.

(2) *Fits:* causes include epilepsy, head injury and cerebral tumour.
(3) *Blackouts:* causes include dysrhythmias, aortic stenosis, pulmonary stenosis, postural hypotension and vasovagal attacks.
(4) *Abnormal sensation and power:* causes include neuropathy, myasthenia gravis and cerebrovascular accident.
(5) *Amnesia after recent head injury:* the patient will require head injury observations. Avoid general anaesthesia if possible; if not, avoid giving drugs which may mask signs of a developing haematoma.

Musculoskeletal system

Stiff joints: beware of intubation problems and difficulty with positioning the patient on the table.

Examination

General

(1) *Abnormal facies:* this is often diagnostic; e.g. congenital abnormalities, endocrine diseases, Parkinson's disease, myasthenia gravis.
(2) *Skeletal abnormalities:* may cause respiratory insufficiency or a difficult intubation. Such patients require careful movement and positioning on the table.
(3) *Obesity:* see Chapter 9.
(4) *Cachexia:* use reduced doses of drugs.
(5) *Weight:* gives a rough guide to drug doses.
(6) *Respiratory insufficiency:* manifests as dyspnoea at rest and inability to complete a sentence in one breath.
(7) *Conjunctivae:* note anaemia.
(8) *Central cyanosis:* causes include ventilation/perfusion abnormality (improved by oxygen), methaemoglobinaemia and sulphaemoglobinaemia (not improved by oxygen).
(9) *Peripheral cyanosis:* causes include cold, heart failure, hypovolaemia, shock, fear and Raynaud's disease.
(10) *Purpura:* causes include old age and bleeding problems.
(11) *Clubbing:* causes include arteriovenous fistula, cyanotic congenital heart disease, chronic suppurative lung disease, bronchial carcinoma, subacute infective endocarditis and cirrhosis. Congenital clubbing is not significant.

(12) *State of veins:* note sites for cannulation. Poor filling is caused by cold, fear or hypovolaemia.
(13) *Dentition:* note any intubation problems and crowns.
(14) *Shape, length and mobility of neck:* note intubation problems with short, fat and/or rigid necks.
(15) *Ability to open mouth:* note any intubation problems.
(16) *Receding chin:* note a possible intubation problem.
(17) *Pyrexia:* consider avoiding atropine and monitor temperature. Look for possible sources of infection.

Cardiovascular system

Pulse

(1) *Character:*
    (a) low volume with normal upstroke: causes include shock, mitral stenosis and pericardial effusion.
    (b) plateau: causes include aortic stenosis and hypertrophic cardiomyopathy.
    (c) collapsing: causes include pyrexia, anaemia, pregnancy, aortic regurgitation, patent ductus arteriosus, arteriovenous fistula and aortic atherosclerosis.
    (d) bisferiens: combined aortic stenosis and regurgitation.
    (e) alternans: is a sign of left ventricular failure.
    (f) paradoxus: occurs in normal patients but if it is exaggerated consider pericardial effusion and constrictive pericarditis.
(2) *Rate:*
    (a) normal range is 60–100 beats per minute.
    (b) bradycardia: causes include physical fitness, drugs, myxoedema and complete heart block.
    (c) tachycardia: causes include pyrexia, thyrotoxicosis, hypovolaemia, myocardial ischaemia, fear and pain.
(3) *Rhythm:* abnormal rhythm requires an ECG for diagnosis.

Blood pressure

(1) *Normal range:* varies with age.
(2) *Hypertension:* causes include renal disease, Cushing's disease, phaeochromocytoma, primary aldosteronism, coarctation and obesity. Serial readings are required before hypertension is diagnosed.

(3) *Hypotension:* causes include hypovolaemia, dehydration and shock.

Internal jugular central venous pressure

(1) *Normal range:* 2–4 cmH$_2$O vertically above the sternal angle when subject reclines at 30° to horizontal.
(2) *Elevated CVP:* causes include right ventricular failure, superior vena caval obstruction, tricuspid valve disease, pericardial effusion, constrictive pericarditis, cardiac tamponade, fluid overload and hyperdynamic circulatory states (e.g. anaemia, arteriovenous fistula, Paget's disease).

Apex beat

(1) *Normal position:* in fifth intercostal space in the mid-clavicular line.
(2) *Displacement:* is due to myocardial hypertrophy or mediastinal displacement.
(3) *Impalpable apex beat:* may be due to obesity, emphysema, pericardial effusion, shock or dextrocardia.

Thrills

The presence of thrills always indicates organic heart disease.

Heart sounds

(1) *Third and fourth heart sounds:* always indicate organic heart disease in patients over 40 years of age.
(2) *An opening snap:* is diagnostic of mitral stenosis.

Murmurs

(1) *All diastolic, continuous and pansystolic murmurs:* indicate significant heart disease.
(2) *Loud systolic murmurs:* may indicate significant disease.
(3) *Soft late systolic murmurs:* are usually benign.

Peripheral oedema

Causes of peripheral oedema include cardiac failure, venous incompetence, deep vein thrombosis, inferior venal caval obstruction, lymphatic obstruction, pre-eclamptic toxaemia, acute glomerulonephritis and low serum proteins.

Allen's test

See p. 22.

ECG

An ECG may show myocardial infarction or ischaemia, dysrhythmias and conduction defects, hypertrophy of individual chambers, pericarditis and electrolyte imbalance. It does not show the mechanical state of the heart.

Respiratory system

Accessory muscles

Use of accessory muscles of respiration indicates severe respiratory insufficiency.

Stridor

Stridor indicates tracheal or laryngeal narrowing.

Presence of protective reflexes

If the cough or laryngeal reflexes are inadequate, the risk of aspiration is increased.

Tracheal deviation

Intubation may be difficult unless the tube is passed in the direction of the deviation.

Shape of chest

Nearly all abnormalities of chest shape result from or cause respiratory insufficiency.

Respiratory rate

(1) *Normal value:* 14 breaths per minute.

(2) *Increased rate:* may be due to respiratory disease, cardiac failure, anxiety, pain, pyrexia, acidosis, hypovolaemia or severe brain damage.

(3) *Decreased rate:* may be due to drug-induced respiratory depression, pain or respiratory failure.

Chest expansion

Place your hands on the patient's chest wall so that the thumbs meet in midline, posteriorly. Ask patient to inspire maximally. Less than 2 cm expansion indicates severe restrictive disease of the lungs or chest wall. Localized diminution of expansion may be due to collapse, consolidation or pleural effusion.

Percussion

(1) *Cardiac and hepatic dullness:* are diminished by emphysema.

(2) *'Stony' dullness:* is caused by a pleural effusion.

(3) *Dullness:* is caused by consolidation, atelectasis or pleural thickening.

(4) *Hyper-resonance:* may be due to pneumothorax or emphysema.

Auscultation

(1) *Diminished breath sounds:* are caused by airway obstruction, pneumothorax, pleural effusion or pleural thickening.

(2) *Bronchial breathing:* is caused by consolidation.

(3) *Rhonchi:* are caused by narrowing of airways. Consider giving preoperative bronchodilators.

(4) *Crepitations:* are caused by pulmonary oedema or secretions. Crepitations due to loose secretions may be dispersed by coughing.

(5) *Pleural rub:* causes include pneumonia and pulmonary embolism.

Chest x-ray

A chest x-ray may confirm the clinical diagnosis. Note the position of the trachea, pneumothorax, pleural effusion, cavitating tuberculosis, bullae and pneumonic changes.

Respiratory function tests

There may be no time for formal tests, and the results rarely give an accurate prediction of the outcome of anaesthesia. Baseline values may, however, be useful postoperatively. The following tests are easy and quick to do:

(1) *Snider match test:* the ability to blow out a match placed 15 cm from the open mouth confirms the absence of severe restrictive or obstructive disease.
(2) *Forced expiratory time test:* the patient expires forcefully after maximal inspiratory effort while the anaesthetist listens through a stethoscope and times the period of expiration. A forced expiratory time of more than 6 seconds indicates moderate or severe obstructive airways disease.
(3) *Arterial blood gases:* normal ranges (breathing air)
    PaO_2 12–15 kPa
    $PaCO_2$ 4.5–6.1 kPa
    $[H^+]$ 36–44 nmol/l
    pH   7.36–7.45
    Standard bicarbonate   21–25 mmol/l

Gastrointestinal system

Abdominal distension

Abdominal distension may splint the diaphragm and cause respiratory insufficiency:

(1) Due to intestinal obstruction: increases the risk of regurgitation and aspiration. Pass a nasogastric tube (see p. 21) and allow to drain freely. Aspirate pre-induction.
(2) Due to a large abdominal mass (e.g. tumour, pregnancy): beware of hypotension due to inferior vena caval compression. The patient should be tilted 15° laterally and allowed to lie supine only when the mass has been removed.

Distended collateral veins

Causes include cirrhosis and chronic inferior vena caval obstruction.

Hepatomegaly

Causes include congestive cardiac failure, early cirrhosis, liver infections, neoplasia and myeloproliferative disorders.

Genitourinary system

Urine volume

(1) *Normal range:* 0.5–1.0 ml/kg per hour.
(2) *Increased volume:* causes include fluid overload, diuretics, diabetes mellitus, diabetes insipidus and the recovery phase of acute renal failure.
(3) *Decreased volume:* causes include hypovolaemia, dehydration, hypotension and renal failure.

Urinalysis

(1) *Protein:* its presence indicates infection or other parenchymal disease.
(2) *Blood:* may be present as a result of trauma or infection of any part of the urinary tract.
(3) *Sugar:* causes include diabetes mellitus, steroids and severe head injury.
(4) *Ketones:* causes include diabetes mellitus, dehydration and starvation.

Nervous system and musculoskeletal system

Muscle tone

(1) *Spasticity and/or clonus:* indicates an upper motor neuron lesion.
(2) *Flaccidity:* indicates a lower motor neuron lesion.
(3) *Cogwheel rigidity:* is typical of Parkinsonism.

Muscle power

The underlying cause of decreased muscle power may be:

(1) *Neurological*—e.g. myasthenia gravis, disseminated sclerosis;
(2) *Muscular*—e.g. muscular dystrophies.

In both types, muscle wasting of recent onset is a contradiction to the use of suxamethonium. Note also the adequacy of respiration and protective reflexes.

Sensation

Areas of diminished or absent sensation should be used for injections and for the insertion of cannulae. These procedures will then be painless.

Valsalva manoeuvre

The patient expires against a closed glottis for 30 seconds. This is normally followed by a fall in blood pressure and an increase in heart rate which is followed in less than 7 seconds by an increase in blood pressure and a decrease in heart rate. If hypotension and tachycardia persist for more than 7 seconds, the autonomic nervous system is abnormal and the patient is likely to be sensitive to rapid postural change and to hypovolaemia. An abnormal response is common in diabetes mellitus.

Conscious level

Causes of decreased conscious level include head injury, epilepsy, drugs, hyperglycaemia, hypoglycaemia, uraemia, myxoedema, hepatic failure, hypoadrenalism, hypopituitarism, electrolyte imbalance, cerebrovascular accidents, septicaemia, hypothermia and hyperthermia.

Size and reactivity of pupils

These should be checked preoperatively, especially in head injuries. If there is any suggestion of abnormality, avoid—if possible—anaesthetic agents which affect pupillary function.

Endocrine system

Thyrotoxicosis, myxoedema, Cushing's syndrome, Addison's disease and acromegaly can often be diagnosed at a glance.

Haematology

Haemoglobin

(1) *Normal values:* male   14–16 g/dl
                     female   12–14 g/dl
(2) *Normal haemoglobin:* may occur in dehydrated but mildly anaemic patients and immediately following acute haemorrhage before resuscitation.
(3) *Anaemia:* if chronic, the blood volume is normal. Preoperative rapid transfusion may cause fluid overload, and the full benefit of increased oxygen-carrying capacity will not be achieved for 24–48 hours. In an emergency, there is no point in delaying the operation until the haemoglobin is normal. Replace blood loss with whole blood and correct the anaemia postoperatively with packed red cells. During the operation and postoperatively give 40% oxygen. If there is no blood loss at the time of the transfusion, 1 unit of whole blood or 250 ml of packed cells will raise the haemoglobin of a 70 kg man by 1 g. Remember that cyanosis due to hypoxia will appear later in anaemic patients.
(4) *Polycythaemia:* is associated with an increased incidence of thrombosis and pulmonary embolism. If time permits, consider venesection. Replace the volume removed with human plasma protein fraction or a blood substitute.

Packed cell volume (PCV)

(1) *Normal values:* male   0.47
                     female   0.42
(2) *Normal PCV:* can occur when dehydration complicates anaemia.
(3) *Increased PCV:* causes include dehydration and polycythaemia.
(4) *Decreased PCV:* causes include anaemia and haemodilution.

Clotting studies

(1) *Coagulation time* in glass. Normal range: 3–11 minutes. A prolonged coagulation time is an indication for more specific tests.
(2) *Prothrombin time.* Normal range: 12–14 seconds, but compare with your own laboratory standard. If prolonged, it may

be due to deficiencies of factors I, II, V, VII or X or to oral anticoagulant therapy. Correct with fresh-frozen plasma or a specific factor concentrate.

(3) *Partial thromboplastin time.* Normal range: 50–100 seconds, but compare with your own laboratory standard. If prolonged, it may be due to deficiency of factors I, II, V, VIII, IX, X, XI or XII or to heparin therapy. Correct with fresh-frozen plasma or specific concentrates.

(4) *Platelets.* Normal range: 150–400 × 10^9/l. If the level is below 50 × 10^9/l, transfuse 6 packs of platelet concentrate immediately prior to induction. If the level is 50–150 × 10^9/l, proceed with the operation and consider transfusing platelets if bleeding is difficult to control.

(5) *Bleeding time.* Normal range: 0–7 minutes. If the bleeding time is prolonged, the cause may be due to any of the above or to capillary fragility.

(6) *Hess test for capillary fragility.* Draw a circle 2.5 cm in diameter on the flexor aspect of the forearm and note any skin blemishes. Apply a tourniquet to the upper arm and inflate to 80 mmHg for 5 minutes. Count the purpuric lesions within the circle. If there are more than 10, capillary fragility is greater than normal. If abnormal bleeding occurs at operation and there is no other cause, ethamsylate 0.75–1.0 g IM or IV may reduce capillary fragility.

Sickledex test

This should be done on all negro patients. If it is positive, they should be treated as described for sickle cell disease (see Chapter 9).

Biochemistry

Serum sodium

(1) *Normal range:* 135–145 mmol/l.

(2) *Low sodium:* due either to sodium loss which is usually associated with dehydration or to overhydration which, if severe, causes cerebral oedema.

(3) *Raised sodium:* due either to dehydration or to overtransfusion with normal saline. It also occurs in head injury and with steroid therapy.

Serum potassium

(1) *Normal range:* 3.6–5.5 mmol/l.
(2) *Low potassium:* causes include vomiting, nasogastric aspiration, diarrhoea, Cushing's disease, hyperaldosteronism and diuretics. Severe potassium depletion is accompanied by a metabolic alkalosis.
(3) *Raised potassium:* causes include renal failure, adrenal insufficiency, trauma and myeloproliferative disease.

Serum urea

(1) *Normal ranges:* 2.5–6.5 mmol/l.
(2) *Low urea:* not clinically important.
(3) *Raised urea:* causes include renal failure, dehydration and diuretics.

Blood glucose

(1) *Normal ranges:* fasting   3.0–5.8 mmol/l.
                        postprandial   <10 mmol/l.
(2) *Low glucose:* give 25 g 50% dextrose IV.
(3) *Raised glucose:* suspect diabetes mellitus (see Chapter 9).

Serum calcium

(1) *Normal range:* 2.12–2.62 mmol/l.
(2) *Raised calcium:* occurs with hyperparathyroidism, multiple myeloma, carcinomatosis, osteoporosis, milk-alkali syndrome, sarcoidosis, acromegaly, Cushing's syndrome and Paget's disease.
(3) *Decreased calcium:* occurs in hypoparathyroidism, pseudohypoparathyroidism, rickets, malabsorption and acute pancreatitis.

Blood gases

(1) *Normal values:* see p. 11.
(2) *Respiratory acidosis* (typically $[H^+]\uparrow$, $Pa_{CO_2}\uparrow$, SB→): due to respiratory insufficiency. If it is severe, ventilate the patient and then treat the specific causes—e.g. chest infection, relative overdose of narcotic analgesics.

(3) *Metabolic acidosis* (typically $[H^+]\uparrow$, $Pa_{CO_2}\downarrow$ or $\rightarrow$, SB$\downarrow$): treat the cause—e.g. diabetes mellitus, hypoxia, renal failure, amino acid infusion. If the acidosis is severe and myocardial depression occurs, give sodium bicarbonate according to the formula:

Volume 8.4% sodium bicarbonate (ml) =

$$\frac{\text{Base deficit} \times 0.3 \times \text{body weight (kg)}}{2}$$

Repeat if necessary after 1 hour, having checked gases and used the formula to calculate the dose.

(4) *Respiratory alkalosis* (typically $[H^+]\downarrow$, $P_{CO_2}\downarrow$, SB$\rightarrow$): treat the cause—e.g. pain, fear.

(5) *Metabolic alkalosis* (typically $[H^+]\downarrow$, $Pa_{CO_2}\rightarrow$, SB$\uparrow$): causes include severe vomiting which should be treated by electrolyte replacement, citrate metabolism following large blood transfusions for which treatment is not required, and potassium deficiency.

(6) *Mixed abnormalities:* may occur as a result of compensatory mechanisms.

Correction of fluid and electrolyte imbalance

Dehydration

Replace water losses with 5% dextrose solution until the hourly urine output is 1 ml/kg. The infusion rate will depend on the age and fitness of the patient: young, fit patients will tolerate 1 litre per hour; old patients with heart disease will only tolerate slower infusion rates. CVP monitoring will help to give warning of imminent overload.

Overhydration

Fluid restriction is sufficient treatment in patients without cerebral oedema. If, however, cerebral oedema is present, give mannitol 1 g/kg as a 20% solution over 30 minutes and then restrict water intake.

Dehydration with sodium loss

Replace fluid and sodium losses with physiological saline solution. Monitor urine output and serum sodium. Severe hyponatraemia may cause delayed recovery from anaesthesia.

Overhydration with sodium chloride solution or sodium retention

Stop the saline infusion and give frusemide 20 mg IV. Excess water in relation to sodium may be lost. Replace with 5% dextrose solution.

Hypokalaemia

If the serum potassium is greater than 3 mmol/l, 100–200 mmol potassium will be required to raise the serum level by 1 mmol/l. If the serum potassium is less than 3 mmol/l, there is often a metabolic alkalosis and more than 200 mmol potassium will be required to replace the loss.

Potassium chloride may be given in normal saline and transfused at a maximum rate of 20 mmol per hour. Monitor the serum potassium to assess progress. If life-threatening dysrhythmias occur, check that hypokalaemia is the only possible cause (see pp. 132–134), and give 5 mmol potassium chloride over 5 minutes into a central vein. Concentrated potassium chloride should never be injected into a peripheral vein. Monitor the ECG and stop injecting if dysrhythmias or peaked T waves occur.

Prior to anaesthesia, serum potassium should be raised to at least 3.5 mmol/l. Even at this level beware of dysrhythmias with halothane and increased sensitivity to depolarizing muscle relaxants.

Hyperkalaemia

Suxamethonium is contraindicated if the serum potassium is greater than 5.5 mmol/l. Several methods of treatment are available:

(1) For emergency but brief reduction in serum potassium, give 20 ml 10% calcium gluconate IV.
(2) Glucose 50 g with 24 units soluble insulin IV stat. will produce a rapid decrease in serum potassium which lasts several hours.

(3) Sodium polystyrene sulphate (Resonium-A) 30 g in methyl-cellulose given as an enema and retained for 9 hours will reduce serum potassium over several hours.
(4) Peritoneal dialysis.
(5) Haemodialysis.

Hypocalcaemia

To correct hypocalcaemia, give 10% calcium chloride 10 ml slowly IV.

Hypercalcaemia

Hypercalcaemia may be corrected by giving trisodium edetate 70 mg in 500 ml 5% dextrose solution over 2–3 hours. If this dose is not adequate, it is unsafe to give a further infusion until the next day. Hydrocortisone 100 mg IV reduces the serum calcium in some cases.

Blood loss

If possible, replace blood loss with cross-matched whole blood. If blood has not been cross-matched, give human plasma protein fraction,, dextran 70 or Haemaccel. Aim to keep the estimated packed cell volume above 0.25. This may involve giving non-cross-matched blood as well as colloid solutions. When giving non-cross-matched blood, try to give blood of the patient's own group; if this is not known or not available, give O-negative blood. Monitor visible blood loss, pulse rate, blood pressure, CVP and urine output. When normal values are reached, the patient may still be vasoconstricted peripherally. Give increments of chlorpromazine IV up to a total dose of 50 mg and transfuse until the CVP returns to normal.

Blood should be filtered and, if possible, warmed.

Plasma loss

Replace with human plasma protein fraction, dextran 70 or Haemaccel, monitoring pulse rate, BP, CVP and urine output. Typically, plasma loss occurs in septicaemic shock, burns and some intestinal conditions. The loss is, therefore, difficult to estimate visually.

Treatment of shock

(1) Give oxygen to maintain the PaO_2 above 9 kPa. If this cannot be achieved with oxygen via a face mask, ventilate the patient. IPPV should be avoided if possible because hypotension will be aggravated.

(2) Replace fluid, monitoring BP, CVP and urine output. Use human plasma protein fraction for septicaemic shock and whole blood for haemorrhagic shock.

(3) Correct metabolic acidosis if $[H^+]$ is greater than 56 nmol/l (pH 7.25). Use the formula to calculate the dose of sodium bicarbonate (see p. 17).

(4) If hypotension does not respond to fluid replacement and correction of metabolic acidosis, give methylprednisolone 30 mg/kg IV over 20 minutes.

(5) In septicaemic shock, take blood for culture. Then give cefuroxime 1.5 g and metronidazole 500 mg IV.

(6) For myocardial failure, give digoxin (see p. 22).

(7) Persistent hypotension requires treatment with a dopamine or isoprenaline infusion.

Management of the full stomach

Before inducing anaesthesia, the patient should be starved for *at least* 6 hours after a full meal and 4 hours after a drink, except, of course, in life-threatening circumstances. Less time is required if only a small amount of water or squash has been taken. Remember that anxiety, pain, alcoholic intoxication, opiates, trauma and pregnancy may cause much longer delays in stomach emptying. Intestinal obstruction, pyloric stenosis and paralytic ileus are always associated with large volumes of stomach contents. Even when an attempt has been made to empty the stomach, the anaesthetist should *always* assume that stomach contents are still present.

Having explained the procedure to the patient, the following methods may be employed. Endotracheal intubation is necessary if the protective reflexes are depressed, as vomiting may be induced.

Passing a stomach tube

This is suitable for removing food. Choose a large-bore stomach tube (24 or 26 French gauge) and lubricate it with water-soluble (e.g. K-Y) jelly. Pass the tube gently into the mouth, using a gag if necessary. Advance the tube slowly, encouraging the patient to swallow. Aspirate as much of the stomach contents as possible with the patient lying supine and then on each side in turn. Remove the tube after the stomach has been emptied.

Passing a nasogastric tube

This is suitable for removing liquid stomach contents. Stiffen an 18 or 21 French gauge nasogastric tube by placing it in the freezing compartment of a refrigerator for 10 minutes. Lubricate the tube with water-soluble jelly, and pass it gently through the nose into the pharynx. Encourage the patient to swallow as the tube is advanced into the stomach. Passage into the stomach is made easier if the patient flexes his neck so that his chin touches the chest wall. Aspirate the contents and test for acidity. If in doubt, check the position of the tube with an x-ray. Never force the tube, or it may pass under the pharyngeal mucosa. If the patient has a history of epistaxis, anticoagulant therapy or bleeding diathesis, the tube should be passed orally. The tube should also be passed orally in head-injured patients with a CSF leak through the nose.

Should the tube pass under the pharyngeal mucosa, observe the patient for haematoma or oedema formation. Give ampicillin 500 mg orally or IM four times daily for 5 days to prevent infection. If respiratory obstruction seems imminent, secure the airway with an endotracheal tube.

In the *unconscious* patient, passage of the nasogastric tube is facilitated by first inserting a split nasal endotracheal tube into the oesophagus. A lubricated nasogastric tube is passed through the endotracheal tube which is then removed.

Having passed the nasogastric tube, suck out as much fluid as possible with the patient lying supine and then on each side in turn. Leave the nasogastric tube on free drainage.

Metoclopramide

A dose of 10 mg IV or IM given 1 hour before operation increases the rate of gastric emptying. Atropine is contraindicated after metoclopramide until the airway has been protected.

Ipecacuanha emetic mixture, paediatric

A dose of 10 ml may induce vomiting in some adults but is unpleasant.

Cimetidine

This does not have any effect on stomach emptying or on the acidity of stomach contents already present. However, 300 mg orally 1.5 hours preoperatively will prevent further acid production.

Magnesium trisilicate

Having attempted to empty the stomach, magnesium trisilicate mixture 20 ml orally 1 hour before operation plus 20 ml immediately prior to induction will reduce the acidity of residual stomach contents.

Sodium citrate

An alternative to magnesium trisilicate mixture is 15 ml 0.3 molar sodium citrate.

Emergency digitalization

Emergency digitalization is indicated in patients with severe congestive cardiac failure and in those with atrial fibrillation causing a radial pulse rate of more than 100 beats per minute.

Check that the patient is not already taking digoxin and that the serum potassium is normal. Give 0.5 mg digoxin IV over 5 minutes while monitoring the ECG for dysrhythmias. Reduce the dose for patients with poor kidney function or hypokalaemia. Then give 0.125–0.25 mg IM daily.

Valid consent

The following criteria must be met.

(1) The patient must be aged at least 16 years. If the patient is less than 16 years old, consent must be obtained from a parent or guardian. If consent is refused, the local authority may grant a Care and Protection Order on the grounds of wilful parental neglect. Never delay an urgent life-saving operation in order to obtain consent.

(2) A truthful explanation of the operation and anaesthetic has been given. The explanation should be tailored to the patient's intelligence and education. There is no need to go into elaborate detail but the patient should be given the opportunity to ask questions. Alternative or additional procedures, if anticipated, should be written on the consent form.

(3) The patient's mental condition should be such that he understands the implications of consent. If the patient cannot consent, a relative or person acting on behalf of the hospital authority may do so.

(4) Consent is not valid if it is given under the influence of drugs, alcohol or premedication.

(5) Jehovah's Witnesses must sign a release form if they do not wish to have a blood transfusion. If this is refused, the anaesthetist should follow his conscience but is under no obligation to treat the patient.

(6) Verbal consent is acceptable but does not provide a written record.

Other legal problems

Administration of dangerous drugs to addicts

It is acceptable to administer dangerous drugs for the relief of pain due to organic disease without notifying the Chief Medical Officer of the Home Office.

Organ removal for transplantation

If the patient dies in hospital, the person lawfully in charge of the body (i.e. a member of the Hospital Management Committee) can give permission for removal of organs. However, every effort should be made to get permission from the patient's next of kin. Organs are rarely removed without the permission of the next of kin even though this is legally permissible. If applicable, two senior doctors independent of the transplant team should have certified brain stem death, using the criteria laid down by the Royal College of Physicians.

Following advice from your consultant

Advice from your consultant should always be followed as he is legally responsible for your actions. However, you also are responsible for your actions. If you sincerely believe that you have been given the wrong advice you may ignore it. It is sensible tactfully to ask another consultant for his opinion before disregarding advice already given.

Premedication

Explanation

A brief explanation of preoxygenation, procedures to be carried out before the patient is asleep and induction of anaesthesia should be given. Try to appear calm and confident while giving the explanation. Allow the patient to ask questions, and answer as clearly and truthfully as possible. If the patient asks questions of a surgical nature which you are unable to answer, refer him to the surgeon and check that he has received a satisfactory answer before inducing anaesthesia. Reassure the patient about postoperative pain and tell him how you plan to relieve it. If a period of postoperative care in the ITU is planned, inform the patient and explain any special procedures such as ventilation in simple terms (e.g. the machine will breathe for you to give your lungs a rest).

Premedicant drugs

These may be unnecessary if you have gained the patient's confidence by your explanation. If drugs are required, a small dose of your usual agent should be used (e.g. diazepam 5–10 mg). Unless there is a specific contraindication (e.g. head injury or respiratory insufficiency), narcotic analgesics should always be given for preoperative pain relief. The dose of induction agent should then be reduced. If ketamine is to be used, lorazepam 2–4 mg orally or IM and atropine 0.6 mg IM 1 hour preoperatively are mandatory.

Subcutaneous heparin

Heparin is indicated for patients on the oral contraceptive pill and for those with a history of deep vein thrombosis or pulmonary embolism. Give heparin 5000 units SC 2 hours before operation.

Antibiotics for patients with heart murmurs or artificial heart valves

Various regimens are used. Use the routine laid down in your hospital or the following.

(1) *Dental, oral and nasal operations:* benzylpenicillin 1 g plus gentamicin 80 mg IM 2 hours preoperatively. If the patient is allergic to penicillin, substitute erythromycin 1 g IM.
(2) *Gastrointestinal and genitourinary operations:* ampicillin 1 g plus gentamicin 80 mg IM 2 hours preoperatively. If the patient is allergic to ampicillin, substitute vancomycin 500 mg IV as an infusion over 20 minutes.

Antibiotic cover should be continued postoperatively.

Steroid cover

To be on the safe side, give cover to all patients who have been on steroids in the previous 2 years. Cover should also be given to patients who have had an adrenalectomy or hypophysectomy.

(1) *Major surgery:*
    1 hour preoperatively   100 mg hydrocortisone IM
    During the operation   100 mg hydrocortisone IV in 500 ml 5% dextrose
    Postoperatively for 3 days   100 mg hydrocortisone IM 6-hourly
    Then reduce dose over the next few days.
(2) *Minor surgery:*
    1 hour preoperatively   100 mg hydrocortisone IM
    Postoperatively for 24 hours   100 mg hydrocortisone IM 6-hourly

Then reduce dose over the next 2 days.
(3) *Brief procedures:*
100 mg hydrocortisone IM 1 hour preoperatively is sufficient.

NB. If hydrocortisone has been omitted in premedication, give 100 mg hydrocortisone IV at induction.

Jaundiced patients

Check the prothrombin time, and if it is prolonged give 4 units of fresh-frozen plasma preoperatively. Vitamin K is unsuitable for emergency cases as it takes too long to become effective.

Patients on MAOIs

See Chapter 9.

Safe sites for intramuscular injections

(1) Deltoid muscle: suitable for small volumes.
(2) Mid-thigh into the vastus externus.
(3) Right buttock: using your left hand, place your index finger on the anterior superior iliac spine, middle finger on the iliac crest and palm flat on the skin. Inject in the triangle between the fingers in order to avoid the sciatic nerve. Use the right hand for the left buttock.

3

Monitoring techniques

Vigilant monitoring is mandatory at all times. Record your observations sequentially. Seek explanations for all changes and, when necessary, give appropriate treatment.

General observation

Observe any part of the patient which can be exposed without contaminating the operating field. The most useful sites are the head, hands, feet and the wound.

(1) *Colour:* look for pallor and cyanosis. Do not be confused by green towels, different lighting and reflection off coloured walls.
(2) *Capillary filling:* blanch the skin with your thumb and note how quickly capillary filling occurs.
(3) *Venous filling:* beware of vasodilator agents which cause distended peripheral veins even though the systemic BP is low.
(4) *Tears and sweating.*
(5) *Rashes.*
(6) *Abnormal bleeding and lack of clot formation.*

Monitoring the cardiovascular system

Pulse

Palpation

Palpation of the radial, carotid, temporal or dorsalis pedis arteries will indicate the presence or absence of a cardiac output. The strength of the palpable pulse gives some indication of the volume of the cardiac output.

Precordial stethoscope

Audible heart sounds indicate only that the heart is pumping. No indication of the volume of the cardiac output is obtained. The waterwheel murmur caused by a large air embolism may also be heard.

Oesophageal stethoscope

This serves the same functions as a precordial stethoscope. It should be positioned in the oesophagus at the level where heart sounds are best heard.

Photoelectric cell

A photoelectric cell attached to the pad of a terminal phalanx: some machines record only pulse rate and give no idea of cardiac output. In others an oscilloscope trace or swinging meter needle gives some indication of changes in the cardiac output. Note that local causes of decreased peripheral blood flow will reduce the amplitude of the pulse, even in the presence of an adequate cardiac output.

Non-invasive blood pressure measurement

Pressure may be measured in the upper arm, thigh or calf. The cuff should cover two-thirds of the length of the upper arm, thigh or calf, and should be at least 20% wider than the diameter of the limb. Inappropriately sized cuffs give inaccurate readings.

Palpation

This requires access to the brachial artery and a cuff on the upper arm. Palpate the brachial pulse and inflate the cuff until the pulse disappears. Deflate the cuff slowly. Note when the pulse reappears. This gives a value for systolic blood pressure which is 10–20 mmHg below values measured by other techniques. Alternatively, the cuff should be placed on the calf or thigh and the dorsalis pedis pulse palpated.

Palpation and auscultation

Estimate the systolic blood pressure using the palpation method. Place the stethoscope over the brachial pulse and inflate the cuff above the estimated systolic pressure. Deflate the cuff slowly. The heart sounds appear at the systolic pressure and become muffled at the diastolic pressure.

Double cuff oscillotonometer

This is useful when direct access to the pulse is difficult. Inflate the cuff to 300 mmHg. Depress the lever and deflate the cuff slowly until maximum deflections of the needle are seen. Release the lever to read the systolic blood pressure. Repeat and note the diastolic blood pressure where the needle stops oscillating. This reading is inaccurate. Automated oscillotonometers are available, but are no more accurate.

Ultrasonic blood pressure monitoring

These devices usually give a digital readout of blood pressure. To obtain an accurate measurement, ensure that the ultrasound emitter is placed directly over the brachial artery.

Invasive blood pressure measurement

Blood pressure may be measured by cannulation of a peripheral artery with good collateral flow or a central artery with a large diameter.

Testing collateral flow to the hand (Allen's test)

(1) Compress the radial and ulnar arteries.

(2) Ask the patient to clench his hand for 3 minutes.

(3) Ask the patient to keep his hand moderately flexed and to open the fist.

(4) If the radial artery is to be cannulated, release the ulnar artery.

(5) The palm of the hand should flush and be a normal colour after 15 seconds. This indicates good collateral flow.

(6) If the ulnar artery is to be cannulated, release the radial artery. The palm should be a normal colour after 15 seconds.

As the radial artery is nearly always dominant, collateral supply is usually good.

Testing collateral flow to the foot

(1) Occlude the dorsalis pedis artery.
(2) Blanch the great toe nail by pressing firmly on the nail bed.
(3) Release pressure on the nail bed. If the nail bed flushes within 10 seconds, the posterior tibial artery collateral circulation is adequate.

Cannulating the radial artery

(1) Use the non-dominant side if possible.
(2) Check the collateral circulation.
(3) Scrub up and wear sterile gloves.
(4) Clean the forearm and hand with a suitable solution (see Appendix 2) and drape with sterile towels.
(5) Immobilize the forearm and hand with the wrist hyperextended and the thumb abducted. Extreme hyperextension of the wrist should be avoided as the radial pulse may become impalpable.
(6) Palpate the course of the artery with first and middle fingers of the left hand. Raise a skin weal with 1% plain lignocaine over the artery.
(7) Make a small skin incision with a blade.
(8) Advance a 20 gauge Teflon parallel-sided cannula through the incision at an angle of 30° to the skin until a brisk flow of bright red blood is observed. The technique is neater if a 2 ml syringe is attached to the cannula which is advanced until blood is aspirated freely.
(9) Grip the needle firmly with the right hand and lower the cannula so that it is nearly parallel to the skin. Then, with the left hand, slide the cannula off the needle into the artery.
(10) Remove the needle and check for free blood flow through the cannula.
(11) Stem the blood flow by pressing on the artery proximal to the cannula and attach a flushing system to the cannula via a Luer lock. The entire flushing system is filled with physiological saline solution containing 5000 units/l preservative-free heparin and is pressurized to 300 mmHg. The complete system consists of the arterial cannula connected via a

narrow-bore extension tube to the flushing device which is in turn connected via a three-way tap to the transducer for measuring blood pressure. If arterial blood samples are to be taken, a three-way tap should be inserted somewhere between the cannula and the flushing device.
(12) Spray the puncture site with tincture of benzoin.
(13) Fix the cannula firmly with adhesive tape. If the cannula has an injection port, this should be occluded with adhesive tape.
(14) Label the dressing with the word 'artery'.

Problems cannulating the radial artery

(1) *Inability to cannulate the artery:* try cannulating other arteries. If this fails, cut down onto the artery and cannulate under direct vision.
(2) *Inability to slide the cannula off the needle into the artery:* this problem may be due to poor positioning of the cannula so that the bevel of the needle is not completely in the arterial lumen. Reinsert the needle and cannula and check that *maximal* free blood flow is obtained before an attempt is made to slide the cannula off the needle. The problem also occurs if the artery is tortuous. Try using the Seldinger technique and pass a thin, sterile guide wire through the needle. Remove the needle and cannula, and then thread the cannula over the guide wire into the artery.
(3) *Cannulation of periarterial tissues:* withdraw the cannula until blood flows freely through it. Advance the cannula briskly. It may pass into the artery.
(4) *Loss of the arterial pulse:* if the artery has been perforated but cannulation has not succeeded and the cannula and needle have been withdrawn, it is vital to prevent haematoma formation. To do this, press firmly on the artery for at least 4 minutes, or until bleeding has stopped, before making another attempt to cannulate the artery. Sometimes after this procedure the arterial pulse is impalpable: arterial spasm has occurred. Spasm usually resolves in 10–20 minutes.

Cannulating the dorsalis pedis artery

Plantarflex the foot and cannulate the artery using the same technique as for radial artery cannulation (see p. 30). Cannulate the artery as distally as possible so that the cannula does not cross the ankle joint. Systolic pressure measured in the dorsalis pedis artery is 5–20 mmHg higher than the equivalent pressure measured in the radial artery.

Cannulating larger arteries

(1) *The axillary artery:* may be cannulated using the technique described on p. 30. The cannula used should be at least 5 cm long. Avoid this site if possible because bacterial contamination of the cannula is likely and fixation is difficult.

(2) *The femoral artery:* is easy to cannulate using a needle, Seldinger guide wire and 13 cm cannula. The risk of infection is greatly increased because of the proximity of the perineum.

(3) *The brachial artery:* may be cannulated using the technique described on p. 30. However, should a clot form on the cannula, circulation to both the ulnar and radial arteries might be impaired.

Problems with the flushing system and readout

(1) *Damped trace:* may be caused by blood in the system, which can be removed by flushing. Air bubbles can also cause damping and are removed by flushing. The system may need to be disconnected to avoid flushing air into the patient. Rarely, radial and dorsalis pedis arteries go into spasm, causing a damped trace. This may be relieved by injecting 10 ml 1% plain procaine or papaverine 10–40 mg diluted in 2–5 ml of Ringer–lactate solution into the artery.

(2) *Blood flow back along the system:* is due to loss of pressure. Check and tighten all connections.

(3) *Unexpectedly low radial artery pressure:* is detected by comparing with the radial artery pressure in the other arm. It may be due to thoracic outlet syndrome or sternal retractors. If due to the former, cannulate another artery and use this for blood pressure measurement.

(4) *Increased pressure which does not fall appropriately after flushing:* may be due to electrical drift which can be corrected by recalibration, or clot formation which requires replacement of the appropriate part of the system. It is best to replace the whole system, taking special care to see that the new system is correctly heparinized.

Electrocardiogram (ECG)

Positioning electrodes

(1) For routine monitoring in fit patients a back plate may be used. Its usefulness is limited because it can be used only in supine patients who do not have spinal deformities. There is no choice of lead. The ECG trace is of low amplitude and may be lost if fluid gets onto the plate.

(2) When it is particularly important to detect changes in the QRS complex and ST segment, place the leads as follows:
   (a) Reference electrode (right arm) on the manubrium sterni.
   (b) Exploring electrode (left arm) in the fifth intercostal space at the anterior axillary line.
   (c) Earth electrode (right leg) on the left shoulder. Set the monitor to lead I.

(3) P waves are seen best by attaching the electrodes to both arms and the right leg. Set the monitor to lead II.

Failure to obtain a clear trace

(1) *Excess baseline excursion:* may be due to one or more loose electrodes or to the location of electrodes on fatty tissue. It may also be due to electrostatic interference from the diathermy; ask the surgeon to use the diathermy in short bursts.

(2) *Small-amplitude QRS complexes:* may be due to a thick chest wall or to disease (e.g. pericardial effusion, myocarditis, cardiomyopathy, myxoedema and emphysema). Other causes include poor contact of the leads, ECG gain control turned down too low, incorrect positioning of electrodes, poor connection of the electrodes to the cable and a broken lead.

(3) *Excess artefact:* causes include loose or dry electrodes (if jelly is required) and electrostatic interference from the diathermy. In the latter instance, ask the surgeon to use the diathermy in short bursts.

(4) *Thick 'noisy' baseline:* is often caused by AC interference. Try plugging the monitor into another socket. Other causes include loose electrode(s), poor electrode-to-cable or cable-to-monitor connections and a defective monitor.

In the awake patient, movement and shivering may cause a poor ECG trace.

Central venous pressure (CVP)

Methods of measurement

(1) *Oscilloscope display or digital readout.* The cannula is connected via a transducer to the monitor. The complete system, including a flushing device, is the same as that described for arterial pressure measurement (p. 30). The transducer should be levelled using a spirit level, either with the angle of Louis if the patient is supine or with the right atrium if the patient is tilted. It may then be accurately zeroed.

(2) *Water manometer.* The system is flushed with 5% dextrose solution. The zero of the scale is levelled in exactly the same way as a CVP transducer. However, the base of the manometer column should be 10 cm below the zero point to reduce the risk of air embolism if the CVP is very low.

Inserting an internal jugular venous cannula

(1) Lie the patient supine with a 10° head-down tilt. Turn his head away from the side of the injection. Place a small pad under his shoulders so that the angle of the jaw, skin of the neck and clavicle are all in the same plane. The anaesthetist stands behind the patient's head.

(2) Scrub up and wear sterile gloves.

(3) Clean the patient's skin with a suitable solution (see Appendix 2) and drape with sterile towels.

(4) Use a 14 gauge metal needle with a 13 cm catheter which can be threaded through the needle. Attach a syringe to the needle. Other types of needle and catheter may be preferred and should be used according to the manufacturer's instructions. Many people find the technique described in the following notes easiest.

(5) Palpate the course of the right carotid artery with the first and middle fingers of the left hand.

(6) Raise a skin weal with 1% plain lignocaine 0.5 cm lateral to the carotid artery and as far away from the clavicle as possible. This depends on where the artery can be palpated but is usually about level with the cricoid cartilage. This step may be omitted if the patient is already anaesthetized.

(7) Make a small skin incision through the bleb.

(8) Advance the needle at right angles to the skin down onto the internal jugular vein, aspirating gently. When the vein has been entered, a 'give' will be felt and dark blood will be aspirated freely. Advance the needle a few millimetres and check that blood can still be aspirated freely. If the needle touches bone, withdraw it, aspirating gently until free blood flow is obtained.

(9) Lower the needle so that it lies almost parallel to the skin and the bevel points caudally. Check that blood can still be aspirated freely.

(10) Remove the syringe and thread the catheter through the needle. Remove the needle and check that blood flows freely from the catheter. If the patient is breathing spontaneously, ask him to breathe in and then out and to continue breathing out while you remove the syringe and attach the flushing system. This prevents air being sucked into the venous system.

(11) Fix the cannula firmly with adhesive tape.

(12) Never withdraw the catheter through the needle.

(13) Check the position of the cannula on a chest x-ray.

Problems associated with internal jugular cannulation

(1) *Failure to hit the vein.* Check the position of the needle in relation to the carotid artery. If it is correctly positioned 0.5 cm lateral to the artery, try directing it a few millimetres more laterally at the next attempt.

(2) *Carotid artery puncture by the needle.* Do not remove the needle until the internal jugular vein has been successfully cannulated lateral to the artery. This prevents the formation of a haematoma which hampers cannulation of the vein. When the vein has been cannulated, remove the needle in the artery and apply firm pressure to the puncture site for at least 5 minutes or until bleeding has stopped.

(3) *Pneumothorax/haemothorax.* If the needle is advanced at right angles to the skin, these problems should not occur. If they do, insert a chest drain and connect it to an underwater drain.

(4) *Chylothorax.* This is a complication of left-sided cannulation and may require insertion of a chest drain.

Cannulation of the basilic vein in the cubital fossa

(1) Position the arm in moderate abduction with the elbow in the neutral position. Turn the patient's head towards the side being cannulated.
(2) Apply a tourniquet above the elbow.
(3) Use sterile technique.
(4) Choose a catheter at least 60 cm long. The Drum cartridge catheter is the most suitable.
(5) Raise a skin bleb with 1% lignocaine in a suitable position for cannulation of the basilic vein, which should be visible or palpable on the ulnar side of the arm.
(6) Advance the needle through the bleb into the basilic vein, looking for blood flow into the catheter. When blood flow is seen, advance the catheter into the vein as described on the instructions with each cartridge.
(7) If the catheter sticks in the axilla, try abducting the arm to 90°.
(8) Check the position of the catheter on a chest x-ray. If it has passed into the neck, withdraw it so that the tip lies in the thoracic cavity. Passage into the neck should be suspected if neck compression raises the CVP by more than 10 cmH_2O.
(9) If you fail to cannulate the basilic vein, it is worthwhile trying to cannulate the cephalic vein. It may, however, be impossible to pass the catheter further than the point where the vein enters the clavipectoral fascia.
(10) *Never* withdraw the catheter through the needle. If withdrawal is necessary, remove catheter and needle together.

Cannulation of the subclavian vein

(1) Lie the patient supine with a 10° head-down tilt. Turn the head away from the side of the injection. The arms should be placed by the patient's side with the shoulders relaxed. The anaesthetist stands beside the patient, on the side of the injection.
(2) Scrub up and wear sterile gloves.
(3) Clean the skin with a suitable solution (see Appendix 2) and drape with sterile towels.
(4) Use a 14 gauge needle and a 10–15 cm catheter which will pass through it. Attach a syringe to the needle. As for

internal jugular cannulation, other types of needles and cannulae are available and should be used according to the manufacturer's instructions.

(5) Palpate the acromioclavicular and sternoclavicular joints and estimate the mid-point of the clavicle.

(6) Raise a skin bleb with 1% plain lignocaine at least one finger's breadth below the lower border of the mid-point of the clavicle. Infiltrate also the subcutaneous tissues in a line from the skin bleb towards the sternal notch until the lower border of the clavicle is reached.

(7) Advance the needle through the skin bleb towards the sternal notch until the clavicle is felt.

(8) Withdraw the needle slightly and step it down the clavicle until it slips under the lower border of the clavicle.

(9) Advance the needle under the clavicle towards the sternal notch, aspirating gently until blood flows freely into the syringe.

(10) Remove the syringe and advance the catheter through the needle into the subclavian vein. Remove the needle. Check that blood flows freely down the catheter. If the patient is breathing spontaneously, ask him to take a breath in and then out and to continue breathing out until you have removed the syringe and attached the flushing system.

(11) Stitch the catheter in place, cover with several gauze swabs and fix with adhesive tape.

(12) Check the position of the catheter on a chest x-ray. If it has passed into the head, withdraw it until it lies in the thoracic cavity.

Problems associated with subclavian vein cannulation

(1) *Failure to hit the vein.* Slight variations in anatomy may be the cause. Try aiming the needle slightly higher above the sternal notch.

(2) *Puncture of the subclavian artery.* Withdraw the needle and direct it slightly more superficially. Usually there is very little problem from arterial puncture. Rarely, a haemothorax requires draining.

(3) *Pneumothorax/haemothorax.* Insert a chest drain and attach it to an underwater seal.

(4) *Chylothorax.* This is a complication of cannulation of the left subclavian vein and may require a chest drain.

Monitoring the respiratory system

Auscultation

Check that both sides of the chest are being inflated equally following intubation and that there are no abnormal breath sounds during anaesthesia.

Tidal volume and minute volume

Measure with a Wright's respirometer.

Inflation pressure

This can be measured if the patient is being ventilated with a ventilator incorporating a pressure gauge.

Blood gases

See p. 11.

Oxygen analyser

An oxygen analyser incorporated into the anaesthetic circuit is a useful safety feature.

End-tidal carbon dioxide monitor

This is useful for assessing the adequacy of ventilation and as a sensitive detector of air embolism. The normal value is 4.5–6 kPa.

Temperature monitoring

Core temperature

The normal range is 36.9–37.7°C. Measure as follows:

(1) *Using an oesophageal probe* placed in the lower fourth of the oesophagus. If correctly placed, this gives a rapid accurate measurement of core temperature. The probe is passed by the method used for nasogastric tubes (p. 21). It should never be forced.

(2) *Using a rectal probe*. These probes respond slowly because they tend to become covered in faeces.
(3) *Using a thermometer* placed in the axilla with the arm abducted. The temperature recorded is 1°C lower than that measured in the oesophagus.

Skin temperature

This may be measured by attaching a skin probe to the pad of the great toe or third finger.

Urine output

Measure urine output accurately by catheterizing the patient and collecting urine hourly. Normal urine output is usually 0.5–1 ml/kg per hour.

Blood loss

Visual estimation

This method is very inaccurate. Four large blood-soaked abdominal swabs very roughly represent 500 ml blood loss; 2 litres of blood covers approximately 1 m^2 of floor. The volume of blood in the suction bottle should also be noted, remembering that it may be mixed with other fluids.

Colorimetric estimation

The swabs are washed in a known volume of water. The haemoglobin content of the water is measured in a colorimeter and, provided the patient's haemoglobin is known, the blood loss can then be estimated.

Gravimetric estimation

This method can only be used if the surgeon uses dry swabs of known weight to mop up the blood. The swabs are weighed after use and the difference from the dry weight is calculated; 1 ml of blood weighs 1 g. Inaccuracies occur if the swab is wetted by other fluids.

Intracranial pressure monitoring

Normal intracranial pressure in the supine patient is 6–15 cmH$_2$O. In the rare event that the intracranial pressure is being monitored during non-cranial surgery, the anaesthetist should note the pressure and use a technique designed to reduce it (see Chapter 8). During craniotomies the state of the brain will be visible.

Monitoring blood chemistry

Serum potassium, sugar and acid–base status should be monitored in some cases (see Chapter 9). Alert the laboratory preoperatively.

What and when to monitor

Deciding what to monitor is largely a matter of common sense. General observations, auscultation following intubation, pulse and non-invasive blood pressure monitoring should be routine for all cases. Other forms of monitoring will depend on the case. Reference to Chapter 9 and the use of the following lists give a rough guide to the parameters which should be monitored.

Invasive blood pressure monitoring

Use this for patients where there may be minute-to-minute changes in blood pressure or where other anaesthetic activities preclude frequent BP measurement by indirect techniques. Patients with this type of problem often also require repeated blood gas analysis, and this is another indication for arterial cannulation.

Electrocardiogram (ECG)

This should be used for all but the briefest minor cases. The back plate is adequate if the patient is fit and ECG changes are unlikely to occur. If dysrhythmias are anticipated, the leads should be positioned so that the P wave is clearly visible (see p. 33). If ischaemia is anticipated, position the leads so that the QRS complex and ST segment are seen best (see p. 33).

Central venous pressure (CVP)

The CVP should be monitored in all cases where large volumes of fluid may have to be given and for cases where smaller volumes are required but there is a risk of overload.

Tidal volume and minute volume

These should be checked in all ventilated patients.

Inflation pressure

The inflation pressure should be noted when available.

Core temperature

The core temperature should be measured in all pyrexial patients if there is any suspicion that malignant hyperpyrexia is developing and in all patients who are likely to become hypothermic (e.g. during massive blood transfusion or a long operation).

Skin temperature

This should be measured in all patients lying on a warming blanket. The blanket should never be more than a few degrees warmer than the patient's skin or burns may result.

Skin/core temperature difference

A useful measure of peripheral vasoconstriction in hypovolaemic patients, it can be used to monitor the adequacy of fluid replacement, especially in conjunction with CVP monitoring, when vasodilators are given.

Urine output

Urine output is another useful indicator of satisfactory fluid replacement.

Blood loss

Visual blood loss estimation is usually sufficient if assessment of the adequacy of fluid replacement also includes pulse, BP, CVP and skin/core temperature difference measurement. If more accurate estimation is required, the colorimetric method is best. Blood should be mopped up from the floor and included in the calculations. Losses onto the drapes can only be measured after the operation is over.

Blood chemistry

Indications are given in Chapter 9.

Ideally, all monitoring should commence in the anaesthetic room prior to induction of anaesthesia. Pain during insertion of cannulae should be minimized by premedication, local anaesthesia and inhalation of 50% nitrous oxide in oxygen. The last mentioned may induce sleep in frail patients. The anaesthetist should always be on the alert for airway obstruction if the patient falls asleep. The risk may be minimized by asking the patient to hold the mask himself. If he falls asleep, he will let the mask fall away from his face and wake up quickly. Some patients may be unable to tolerate a head-down tilt. It is preferable to anaesthetize these patients before cannulating central veins.

Local anaesthetic techniques

Indications

(1) Any procedure for which local anaesthesia will provide satisfactory operating conditions.
(2) Pulmonary disease provided that the patient will be able to tolerate the position required for the operation.
(3) Previous adverse reaction to general anaesthetic agents.
(4) Anticipated problems with maintaining the airway or intubation.
(5) Urgent operation without adequate starvation. If time is available, it is preferable to starve the patient when large doses of local anaesthetic are to be used because a toxic reaction may cause depression of laryngeal reflexes, hypotension and vomiting.

Absolute contraindications

(1) Refusal by the patient.
(2) Allergy to local anaesthetic drugs.
(3) Infection at the site of injection.
(4) Anticoagulant therapy.
(5) Bleeding diatheses.
(6) Use of adrenaline-containing solutions for patients on tricyclic antidepressants (see Appendix 1). Felypressin-containing solutions are safe for these patients.

Relative contraindications

(1) Lack of patient co-operation.
(2) Neurological disease. An exacerbation may be blamed on the anaesthetic technique.

Local anaesthetic toxicity

Prevention

(1) Never exceed the maximum dose.

	Plain	*With adrenaline*
Bupivacaine	2 mg/kg 4-hourly	2 mg/kg 4-hourly
Lignocaine	3 mg/kg	7 mg/kg
Prilocaine	6 mg/kg	8.5 mg/kg

NB. 1 ml of a 1% solution contains 10 mg.

The maximum dose of adrenaline is 500 µg—i.e. 0.5 ml 1:1000 solution. The concentration of adrenaline should never exceed 1:200000. To achieve a concentration of 1:250000 put 4 drops of 1:1000 adrenaline through a 21 gauge needle into 25 ml anaesthetic solution.
(2) Use the lowest dose and concentration of local anaesthetic which will provide satisfactory operating conditions.
(3) Inject local anaesthetic slowly and aspirate frequently.
(4) Use reduced doses in elderly and debilitated patients.

Signs of toxicity

Central nervous system

Nervousness, tremor and convulsions are followed by respiratory depression and apnoea.

Cardiovascular system

Severe hypotension may be followed by cardiac arrest.

Gastrointestinal system

There may be nausea, vomiting and abdominal pain.

Allergy

A rash, bronchospasm or anaphylactic shock may occur.

Treatment of a toxic reaction

Respiratory depression

Maintain the airway, intubating if necessary; give 100% oxygen and assist or control ventilation.

Convulsions

Give diazepam 0.1–0.2 mg/kg slowly IV
   or paraldehyde 10 ml IM
   or thiopentone 1–2 mg/kg IV slowly plus suxamethonium 1 mg/kg IV.
   Then intubate and ventilate, remembering to take precautions if the stomach is not empty (see p. 82).

Hypotension

Give oxygen via a face mask even if respiration is satisfactory, elevate the legs and give up to 1 litre of human plasma protein fraction, dextran 70 or Haemaccel. If the blood pressure does not rise give ephedrine 15–30 mg IM or metaraminol 1–2 mg IV.

Cardiac arrest

See pp. 127–132.

Preoperative preparation

Preoperative history and examination

See pp. 3–17.

Explanation to the patient

This should include:

(1) A description of the technique, including the position the patient will be required to adopt for administration of the anaesthetic.
(2) Reassurance that the operation will not start until the anaesthetic is effective.
(3) A warning that although the procedure will be painless, the patient may feel touch and pressure.

Premedication

The choice depends on the anaesthetist's personal preference. Some suggestions are:

(1) Diazepam 10–20 mg orally 1 hour preoperatively.
(2) Lorazepam 2–4 mg orally 1 hour preoperatively.
(3) Papaveretum 10–20 mg plus droperidol 5–10 mg IM 1 hour preoperatively.

These may be supplemented during the operation by a mixture of fentanyl 0.1 mg plus droperidol 10 mg made up to 5 ml with water. Give 1 ml increments IV, watching for sedation and signs of overdose (i.e. respiratory depression or hypotension).

Technique common to all local anaesthetics

(1) Prepare resuscitation equipment, which should include the following:
    (a) face mask;
    (b) method for inflating the lungs;
    (c) endotracheal tube;
    (d) laryngoscope;
    (e) oxygen supply;
    (f) diazepam, paraldehyde, thiopentone and suxamethonium;
    (g) suction apparatus and catheters;
    (h) ephedrine and metaraminol;
    (i) standard resuscitation drugs.
(2) Ask the patient to remove any clothing which may contaminate the site of the injection.
(3) Insert an indwelling cannula suitable for injection of drugs and rapid transfusion of fluid.
(4) Position the patient on a table which can be tilted to the head-down position.
(5) Check landmarks and mark the skin.
(6) Scrub up and wear sterile gloves. A gown should be worn if bacterial contamination of the injection site could be hazardous (i.e. epidural and spinal anaesthesia).
(7) Lay out and check the equipment. Also check the contents and concentration of ampoules. Adrenaline should *never* be injected into fingers, toes or other appendages.

(8) Clean the skin with a suitable solution (see Appendix 2), starting at the site of injection and spiralling outwards. Allow the skin to dry.

(9) Drape the patient with sterile towels.

(10) Proceed with a specific technique.

(11) Having completed the anaesthetic, use whatever monitoring techniques you would have considered appropriate for the same patient, had he been having a general anaesthetic. For all techniques except local infiltration, the anaesthetist should remain with the patient for the duration of the operation.

(12) Screen the patient with sterile towels and check that unpleasant reflections are not visible in the theatre light.

(13) Discourage inappropriate conversation amongst the medical and nursing staff. In particular, discourage the surgeon from enquiring if the patient can feel the incision. It will be obvious if the anaesthetic is inadequate.

(14) Allow the patient to sleep during the procedure if he wishes. If he is awake, talk cheerfully and quietly to him. Avoid giving gruesome details about the operation. Be truthful about how long it will take to complete the operation—it may seem even longer to the patient than it does to you.

Infiltration anaesthesia—skin

Indication

Suture of lacerations.

Special equipment

(1) 25 or 23 gauge needle.

(2) 0.25–0.5% lignocaine. Adrenaline may be used except in fingers, toes or other appendages. The volume of anaesthetic used will be variable but should not exceed the maximum safe dose of lignocaine.

Technique

Inject the local anaesthetic into the subcutaneous tissues around the site of the laceration. As far as possible, infiltrate fan-wise around the puncture site. If a second puncture is required, inject into an area which has already been anaesthetized. This method reduces to a minimum the number of painful injections.

Infiltration anaesthesia—fracture haematoma

Indication

Reduction of wrist fractures. Analgesia is often barely adequate. The technique is useful for very frail patients and for the rapid treatment of mass casualties. It should not be used routinely because it converts a closed fracture to an open fracture which may become infected.

Special equipment

(1) 25 or 23 gauge needle at least 2 cm long.
(2) 15 ml 1% plain lignocaine,
    or 15 ml 1% plain prilocaine.

Technique

(1) Clean the skin with special care.
(2) Palpate the fracture.
(3) Inject local anaesthetic slowly into the periosteum and soft tissues around the fracture.

NB. Aspiration of haematoma may be indistinguishable from venous blood. Therefore, inject very slowly and be alert for the first sign of toxicity, which is usually circumoral tingling.

Intravenous regional anaesthesia (Bier's block)

Indications

(1) Operations on the hand, forearm and lower part of the upper arm.
(2) Operations on the lower leg and foot.

Contraindications

(1) Sickle cell disease.
(2) Sickle cell trait.

(3) Sickle cell haemoglobin C disease.
(4) Sickle cell thalassaemia.
(5) Surgery on blood vessels.

Special equipment

(1) Blood pressure cuff or a pneumatic tourniquet.
(2) 20 or 22 gauge plastic cannula. Butterfly needles may be used but have a greater tendency to cut out of the vein when the Esmarch bandage is used.
(4) Esmarch bandage or inflatable splint.
(5) Local anaesthetic:

(a) *Upper limb:*	plain 0.5% prilocaine 40 ml, or plain 0.5% lignocaine 40 ml, or plain 0.2% bupivacaine 40 ml;
(b) *lower limb:*	plain 0.5% prilocaine 60–80 ml, or plain 0.25% lignocaine 50–100 ml.

Technique

(1) Check the systolic blood pressure.
(2) Insert a cannula into the most peripheral vein available.
(3) Place the blood pressure cuff or pneumatic tourniquet on the middle part of the upper limb or thigh over cotton wool padding. Secure it with adhesive tape or cotton bandage.
(4) Exsanguinate the limb with an Esmarch bandage or inflatable splint. If the limb is painful it is sufficient to elevate it for 3 minutes while compressing the brachial or femoral artery.
(5) Inflate the cuff to a pressure of 50–100 mmHg above the systolic BP for the upper limb or 100–150 mmHg above the systolic BP for the lower limb.
(6) Check that the peripheral pulses are absent.
(7) Inject the local anaesthetic solution as a single dose. If the operation site is more peripheral than the cannula, place a second cuff immediately proximal to the cannula prior to injection. When analgesia is present distally, remove this lower cuff, elevate the limb and milk the anaesthetic solution up the limb.
(8) Tourniquet pain almost always occurs after 45–60 minutes. It may be reduced by giving fentanyl 0.05 mg and droperidol 5 mg slowly IV immediately after anaesthesia has been induced. Alternatively, a double cuff may be used: anaes-

thesia is induced with proximal cuff inflated; when the area under the distal cuff is anaesthetized, this cuff is inflated and the upper cuff is then deflated. The double cuff is also safer because if one cuff fails the other can be rapidly inflated.

(9) When the operation is over or after 20 minutes, whichever is the later, the cuff is deflated.

(10) Observe the patient for signs of toxicity for 15 minutes after the cuff has been deflated.

Complications

(1) Inadvertent early deflation of cuff. Treat signs of toxicity if they occur.

(2) Leakage of local anaesthetic through an inadequately inflated cuff. Treat any toxic signs that occur.

(3) Methaemoglobinaemia only occurs with prilocaine. Treat with 1% methylene blue 1 mg/kg IV.

Digital nerve block

Indications

Simple operations on fingers and toes.

Special equipment

(1) 25 gauge needle.
(2) 1% *plain* lignocaine 4 ml per digit,
    or 1% *plain* prilocaine 4 ml per digit,
    or 0.5% plain bupivacaine 4 ml per digit.

Technique

Local anaesthetic 1.5–2 ml is injected down each side of the digit near to the metacarpophalangeal/metatarsophalangeal joint. Inject slowly to minimize pain, and avoid using larger volumes of anaesthetic which may cause mechanical ischaemia.

Supraclavicular brachial plexus block

Indications

Operations on the upper limb and shoulder.

Special equipment

(1) 21 or 23 gauge needle at least 5 cm long.
(2) 1.5% lignocaine with adrenaline 20–30 ml,
   or 0.5% plain bupivacaine 20 ml.
(3) Equipment for insertion of a chest drain.

Technique

(1) Lie the patient supine with his head on a low pillow, turned away from the side of the block. The arms should be placed by the patient's side with the shoulders relaxed. The anaesthetist stands at the head of the table.
(2) Raise a skin bleb with 1% lignocaine 1 cm above and immediately lateral to the mid-point of the clavicle (the mid-point of the clavicle can sometimes be identified by extending an imaginary line towards the clavicle along the course of the external jugular vein; the line crosses the clavicle at its mid-point).
(3) Through the bleb insert the needle at an angle of 80° to the skin and direct it caudally until it touches the first rib.
(4) Move the needle cautiously backwards and forwards along the first rib until the patient feels a tingling sensation in the arm. Withdraw the needle a few millimetres and inject 7–10 ml of local anaesthetic. Repeat until paraesthesia has been elicited in the upper arm, lower arm and both sides of the hand, indicating that all three divisions of the brachial plexus have been located and anaesthetized.
(5) If paraesthesia has not been elicited, step the needle forwards on the first rib until it is as close as possible to the subclavian artery. Inject 8 ml of local anaesthetic. Then step the needle backwards along the first rib, injecting the local anaesthetic as you go.
(6) Following induction of anaesthesia and postoperatively the patient should be observed for signs of pneumothorax which may require treatment with a chest drain, or dislocation of the shoulder which requires reduction. If in doubt, take a chest x-ray to diagnose a pneumothorax.

Axillary brachial plexus block

Indications

Operations on the distal part of the upper limb, forearm and hand.

Special equipment

(1) 21 gauge needle about 5 cm long.
(2) 1.5% lignocaine with adrenaline 25–30 ml,
    or 1.5% prilocaine with adrenaline 25–30 ml,
    or 0.5% plain bupivacaine 30 ml (if necessary reduce the
    concentration to avoid exceeding the maximum dose).

Technique

(1) The patient lies supine with the arm externally rotated and
    abducted at an angle of 90° to the trunk.
(2) Palpate the axillary artery and introduce the needle slightly
    above and directed slightly towards the artery. A 'give' is felt
    as the needle enters the axillary sheath just above the artery.
    The needle oscillates with the arterial pulse.
(3) Apply a tourniquet to the arm just below the axilla. Leave this
    on until anaesthesia is established.
(4) After aspirating, inject the local anaesthetic.

Complication

Puncture of the artery. Press firmly on the artery for 4 minutes to
prevent haematoma formation. The presence of haematoma in
the axillary sheath may prevent the local anaesthetic reaching all
the nerves, resulting in a patchy block.

Spinal anaesthesia

Indications

(1) Low spinal (S1–5) for cystoscopy and operations on the anus,
    penis and scrotum.
(2) Mid-spinal for abdominal operations below the umbilicus,
    operations on the prostate, gynaecological procedures and
    operations on the lower limbs.

Absolute contraindications

(1) Sepsis near or at the site of injection.
(2) Anticoagulant therapy.
(3) Bleeding diathesis.

(4) Hypovolaemia and shock.
(5) Beta-blocker therapy.
(6) Septicaemia.
(7) Fixed cardiac output—e.g. aortic stenosis, constrictive pericarditis, complete heart block.
(8) Raised intracranial pressure.

Relative contraindications

(1) MAOI therapy, because the use of vasopressors to treat
hypotension is contraindicated.
(2) Active neurological disease. An exacerbation may be
blamed on the anaesthetic.
(3) Ischaemic heart disease. Ischaemia may be aggravated by
hypotension.
(4) Scoliosis. It may make administration technically difficult.
(5) Previous laminectomy. It may be possible to inject above or
below the operation site.

Special equipment

(1) 22 or 25 gauge spinal needle.
(2) Sise introducer if a 25 gauge needle is used. A 19 gauge
hypodermic needle is a good substitute for a Sise introducer.
(3) Hyperbaric local anaesthetic solution:
    (a) *low spinal:*   'heavy' 5% lignocaine 1 ml,
                  or 'heavy' 5% prilocaine 1 ml;
    (b) *mid-spinal:* 'heavy' 5% lignocaine 1.5 ml,
                  or 'heavy' 5% prilocaine 1.5 ml.

Preoperative preparation

It is essential to warn the patient about loss of motor power and
reassure him that the paralysis will only be temporary.

Technique

(1) Measure the BP.
(2) Start an infusion of 500 ml normal saline solution to be
completed by the time the local anaesthetic is injected.
(3) Lie the patient in the lateral position with the side to be
operated on lowest.

(4) Having scrubbed up and put on sterile gloves and a gown, prepare the equipment. The local anaesthetic should be drawn up from a sterile ampoule.

(5) Ask your assistant to position the patient. To obtain maximum curvature of the spine, ask the patient to draw his knees as far up to his chest as possible and then to put his chin as near his knees as he is able.

(6) Having cleaned the skin and covered the patient in sterile drapes, palpate the posterior iliac crests through the drapes. The line joining the crests passes through the spine of L4. Palpate the spines of L2 and L3. Then choose the L2–3 or L3–4 interspace.

(7) Anaesthetize the skin and subcutaneous tissues with 1% lignocaine.

(8) Insert the Sise introducer through the skin at right angles to the skin in all directions and then advance it slightly cephalad through the tissues towards the ligamentum flavum.

(9) Insert the spinal needle through the introducer. Note its passage through the ligamentum flavum and epidural space into the subarachnoid space. At all times avoid touching the needle. If it must be handled, use a sterile swab.

(10) When the stilette of the needle is removed, free flow of CSF should be seen. It is often extremely slow if a 25 gauge needle is used. More rapid confirmation of the needle's position is obtained by aspirating CSF with a syringe. If a continuous flow of blood is obtained with the CSF, the procedure should be abandoned. However, if blood-stained CSF rapidly becomes clear, it is safe to continue.

(11) When clear CSF is flowing freely, inject the local anaesthetic solution. Prevent displacement of the needle by holding it between the first finger and thumb with the back of the hand braced against the patient's back.

(12) Withdraw the spinal needle and introducer together, and cover the hole with a small sterile dressing.

(13) *Low spinal.* Sit the patient up for 2 minutes and then lie him flat with the head slightly raised. If a unilateral block is sufficient, lie him on his side with the side to be operated on lowermost.
Mid-spinal. Lie the patient on his back with the knees flexed. Test the level frequently with an ice cube or needle, and if the block is too low tip the patient slightly head down.

NB. Pregnant patients and those with large abdominal tumours should never be allowed to lie supine. Always use a wedge. The wedge may be changed to the opposite side after 5 minutes if a bilateral block is required.

(14) Check the BP frequently for the first 15 minutes. If hypotension occurs, give oxygen and 5 mg increments of ephedrine IV. Pregnant patients should only be given ephedrine in direst circumstances. Transfusion of 1 litre of normal saline or Haemaccel should be sufficient to restore the blood pressure. Do not tip the patient head down for at least 10 minutes after injection of the local anaesthetic. This will increase the level of the block and aggravate hypotension.

Complications

(1) Nausea and vomiting are usually associated with hypotension and will stop when the BP rises. Rarely, prochlorperazine 12.5 mg IM is necessary.

(2) Total spinal. Intubate the patient and ventilate with 100% oxygen until the BP is normal, then 40% oxygen. Treat hypotension with a head-down tilt, ephedrine 5 mg increments IV or a phenylephrine infusion (10 mg in 250 ml physiological saline). Ephedrine 50–100 mg IM is a less effective alternative.

Lumbar epidural anaesthesia

Indications

All operations below the level of the umbilicus. Insertion of an epidural catheter allows additional doses of local anaesthetic to be given during long operations and also provides a route for postoperative pain relief.

Absolute and relative contraindications

These are the same as for spinal anaesthesia (see pp. 52–53).

Special equipment

(1) 17 or 18 gauge Tuohy–Flower needle.

(2) For detecting loss of resistance, either a syringe with an easily movable piston or a Macintosh balloon.

(3) Epidural catheter which has been checked for patency and compatibility with the Tuohy needle.

(4) Bacterial filter.

(5) Local anaesthetic solution:

0.5% plain bupivacaine 1.5–2.5 ml solution per segment to be blocked up to the maximum safe dose; use half this volume in pregnant and elderly patients,

or 0.25% plain bupivacaine 1.5–2.5 ml solution per segment up to the maximum safe dose.

Use of a lower concentration of anaesthetic allows larger volumes to be used without exceeding the maximum dose. Greater spread of anaesthesia is obtained but muscle relaxation is usually unsatisfactory for abdominal operations.

Technique

(1) Allow plenty of time. Up to 1 hour may be needed if an incremental method of inducing anaesthesia is used.

(2) Proceed as for spinal anaesthesia up to 'Technique' item 7 (pp. 52–54).

(3) Nick the skin with a blade.

(4) Insert the Tuohy–Flower needle at right angles to the skin in all directions. Then advance the needle slightly cephalad until it has entered the ligamentum flavum and resistance is felt. This usually occurs about 5 cm below the skin in a patient of normal build. If bony resistance is felt, withdraw the needle slightly, check the alignment of the needle and, if it is correct, walk the needle along the bone until it drops into the ligamentum flavum. If the needle is not correctly aligned, adjust it and proceed as described.

(5) Withdraw the stilette and attach the syringe with the piston withdrawn a little, or the Macintosh balloon and inflate it with air.

(6) Support the needle with the thumb and first finger of the left hand with the back of the hand braced against the patient's back. Advance the needle slowly until resistance is lost. Air will then be injected easily with the syringe, or the balloon will deflate.

(7) Continue to support the needle and check that there is no CSF flowing from it. Advance the catheter down the needle

until the 20 cm mark is at the hub of the needle. If the catheter does not pass freely, try carefully rotating the Tuohy needle through 180°. If this fails, ask the patient to carefully straighten his legs a little. If these manoeuvres fail, remove the needle and catheter together. Never withdraw the catheter through the needle. Start again. If the problem recurs, try another space.

(8) If the catheter passes into the epidural space, withdraw the needle carefully so that the catheter does not come out with it. Then withdraw the catheter so that only 3–5 cm of it remains in the epidural space. The distance from the epidural space to the skin may be estimated by noting the distance the needle was inserted.

(9) Aspirate the catheter.
(a) Free flow of blood indicates catheterization of an epidural vein. Remove the catheter and start again in another intervertebral space.
(b) Aspiration of clear fluid indicates that either the dura has been punctured or local anaesthetic has been injected into the epidural space. Test the fluid with Dextrostix: CSF contains sugar, local anaesthetic does not. If the dura has been punctured, start again in another intervertebral space.

(10) Having satisfied yourself that the catheter is correctly positioned, prime the bacterial filter with local anaesthetic, attach it to the catheter and inject a 2 ml test dose of bupivacaine. Ask your assistant to check the BP frequently and inform you of the results.

(11) Fix the catheter securely so that the injection port lies over one shoulder. Loop the catheter near the injection site before fixing. Any tension on the catheter will not then automatically pull it out.

(12) Ten minutes after the test dose the BP should not have altered and the patient should have normal sensation. It is safe to assume (although not absolute proof) that the dura has not been punctured by the catheter. It is then safe to inject larger doses of anaesthetic. The total dose may be injected at once but you may prefer to inject in 8–10 ml increments, noting the spread of anaesthesia and adjusting the patient's position after each increment. The patient should be tilted in the direction it is desired that the anaesthetic should spread. After each dose of anaesthetic the BP should be checked regularly for 20 minutes.

NB. Pregnant patients and those with large abdominal tumours should never be allowed to lie supine. Always use a wedge. If bilateral anaesthesia is required, inject the local anaesthetic with the patient tipped to one side and after 5 minutes change the wedge to the other side.

(13) Top-ups may be given when the anaesthetic begins to wear off. A top-up may be required after 1 hour but often a much longer period elapses before a top-up is required. The usual dose of anaesthetic for a top-up is 8–15 ml. The BP should be checked regularly for 20 minutes after each top-up.

Complications

(1) Hypotension: manage as for spinal anaesthesia (p. 55).
(2) Total spinal: manage as for spinal anaesthesia (p. 55).
(3) Nausea and vomiting: manage as for spinal anaesthesia (p. 55).
(4) Unilateral block:
    (a) due to the passage of the catheter out through a paravertebral canal. Usually too much catheter has been left in the epidural space. Withdraw the catheter and inject a further dose of local anaesthetic, remembering not to exceed the maximum safe dose;
    (b) due to an epidural septum. You may, if you are very lucky, insert a second catheter into the epidural space on the other side of the septum. It is probably easier to opt for a different anaesthetic technique.
(5) Missed segment. Occasionally the L1 dermatome remains unblocked. To block this area, insert a short-bevelled 21 or 23 gauge needle through the skin at a point two fingers' breadth medial to the anterior superior iliac spine. Advance the needle until it clicks through the external oblique aponeurosis. Inject 0.25% bupivacaine 10 ml under the aponeurosis in a fan-like distribution. Then inject 0.25% bupivacaine 10 ml into the muscle in the same distribution. Do not exceed the maximum safe dose of bupivacaine.
(6) Dural puncture. Having successfully inserted a catheter into another space, proceed with the operation, ensuring that the patient is well hydrated at all times. When epidural anaesthesia is no longer required, infuse 1.5 litres physiological saline solution over 36–48 hours via the epidural catheter in an

attempt to prevent post-lumbar puncture headache. Do not allow the patient to strain at stool, vomit or push during a vaginal delivery.

Further care

Always remove the catheter yourself. Pull gently and check that the catheter is intact. If a portion is retained in the epidural space, inform the patient and consult a neurosurgeon for advice about the necessity for removal.

Anaesthesia for laryngoscopy and intubation

Indications

Awake intubation in patients with active reflexes who are unsuitable for other techniques of intubation.

Contraindications

Severe mucosal damage where rapid absorption of local anaesthetic may occur and cause a toxic reaction.

Cautionary note

If the larynx and trachea are completely anaesthetized, there is a risk of aspiration should regurgitation or vomiting occur. It is preferable, therefore, to anaesthetize only the oral cavity and superior aspect of the larynx, taking care that local anaesthetic does not enter the trachea. This preserves intact tracheal and carinal reflexes. Alternatively, the trachea may be anaesthetized. The patient should not be extubated until the cough reflex has returned.

Premedication

Give atropine 0.6 mg IM 1 hour preoperatively to prevent salivation.

Special equipment

(1) 10 mg benzocaine lozenge.

(2) Dental swabs soaked in 4% plain lignocaine.
(3) 4% lignocaine with adrenaline spray.
(4) 4% lignocaine 2 ml in a syringe attached to a 21 gauge needle.

Do not exceed the maximum safe dose of lignocaine.

Technique

(1) Ask the patient to suck the benzocaine lozenge until it has completely dissolved. This will anaesthetize the mouth and pharynx.
(2) For nasal intubation, spray the nasal cavity with 4% lignocaine with adrenaline. The adrenaline will help to reduce bleeding.
(3) Under direct vision, using a laryngoscope, hold a dental swab soaked in 4% lignocaine in each pyriform fossa for at least half a minute. The swab is most easily held with Krause's forceps.
(4) Intubate the patient with a cuffed tube. Coughing may occur when the tube is placed in the trachea but will resolve when anaesthesia is induced.
(5) To anaesthetize the trachea, clean the skin with an appropriate solution (see Appendix 2). Insert the 21 gauge needle through the cricothyroid membrane into the trachea. Check that air can be freely aspirated. Ask the patient to hold his breath at the end of expiration. Inject 4% lignocaine 2 ml.

Postoperative care after local anaesthesia

Special care for individual techniques is described in the appropriate sections. If any complication has occurred or is suspected, the patient should be detained in hospital until these have been treated or excluded.

After local anaesthesia has worn off, remember that premedication may still be exerting a sedative effect. If the patient is being allowed to go home he should be accompanied and cared for by a relative or friend for at least the next 12–24 hours. The patient should be warned that he should not drive or operate potentially dangerous machinery or domestic equipment for 24 hours.

Even if the patient has not been premedicated, these precautions should still be observed. Although the patient's mental function is normal, he may still faint several hours after local anaesthesia.

5

General anaesthesia

Indications

It is possible to design a general anaesthetic technique to suit each patient. In some patients, local anaesthesia is associated with fewer side effects and is, therefore, preferable. General anaesthesia should be used for all cases where local anaesthesia is contraindicated or unsuitable. Chapter 9 lists conditions which have implications for anaesthesia and should be consulted for possible contraindications.

Local anaesthesia for intubation

See pp. 59–60.

Intravenous agents for induction and intubation

Your choice of intravenous induction agent should be governed by the information in the following section.

Methohexitone sodium (1% solution)

Indications

Methohexitone sodium is the barbiturate induction agent of choice for emergency anaesthesia. It causes less hypotension than thiopentone and recovery is quicker. Although recovery occurs within a few minutes, methohexitone is only metabolized after many hours.

Absolute contraindications

(1) Barbiturate hypersensitivity.
(2) Porphyria.

Relative contraindications

See Chapter 9. Methohexitone should be avoided if possible when it is relatively contraindicated. If it must be used, the dose should be greatly reduced.

Dosage

Give 1–1.5 mg/kg IV depending on whether premedication has been administered. Reduce the dose for patients who are hypovolaemic, dehydrated or frail due to illness or old age.

Complications

(1) Pain on injection. The addition of plain lignocaine 1 mg/ml methohexitone solution reduces the pain.
(2) Apnoea and respiratory depression.
(3) Laryngospasm, coughing and bronchospasm.
(4) Hypotension.
(5) Skeletal muscle activity, reduced by premedication.
(6) Allergy.
(7) Fits.

Complications 2, 3, 4 and 7 may be minimized by injecting slowly.

Thiopentone sodium (2.5% solution)

Indications

Thiopentone may be used in place of methohexitone when methohexitone is not available.

Absolute contraindications

(1) Barbiturate hypersensitivity.
(2) Porphyria.

Relative contraindications

See Chapter 9. If the use of thiopentone is unavoidable, the dosage should be greatly reduced.

Dosage

Give 4–8 mg/kg IV depending on whether premedication has been given. The dose should be reduced to 1–2 mg/kg for hypovolaemic, dehydrated or frail patients.

Complications

(1) Pain which radiates distally from the injection site almost always indicates intra-arterial injection. Stop the injection and treat (see pp. 104–105).
(2) Other complications are similar to those of methohexitone and should be minimized in the same way. Skeletal muscle activity and fits do not occur with thiopentone.

Alphaxalone–alphadolone acetate (Althesin)

Indications

(1) When the barbiturates are contraindicated.
(2) When the patient is to be sent home on the same day as being given the anaesthetic. Althesin is metabolized within minutes of the injection so there is no hangover effect.

Absolute contraindications

(1) Previous adverse reaction to Althesin.
(2) Hepatic failure.

Relative contraindications

(1) Personal or family history of atopy.
(2) Pregnancy.

Dosage

Give 0.05 ml/kg IV slowly. An infusion given at 5–15 ml per hour will provide anaesthesia if a high oxygen concentration is required peroperatively.

Complications

(1) Bronchospasm, laryngospasm and hiccough.
(2) Hypotension.
(3) Anaphylaxis. Bronchospasm and hypotension are very severe.
(4) Dysrhythmias may occur when muscle relaxants are also given.

Etomidate

Indications

As for Althesin (see p. 64).

Absolute contraindication

Previous adverse reaction to etomidate.

Relative contraindication

Pregnancy—safety in pregnancy has not been established.

Dosage

Give 0.3 mg/kg IV slowly. Etomidate is said to have little effect on the cardiovascular system. The author has seen three severe hypotensive reactions which circumstantial evidence suggested were caused by the combination of etomidate and hypovolaemia. It is therefore suggested that the dose of etomidate be reduced for hypovolaemic patients.

Complications

(1) Pain on injection: this may be minimized by injecting into a large vein.
(2) Spontaneous muscle movement: this may be minimized by premedication with narcotic analgesics.

Ketamine

Indications

Ketamine should be considered for patients with cardiovascular instability because it raises the BP. In spite of this advantage, its use is deplored by some anaesthetists because of the high incidence of emergence hallucinations which occur even in premedicated patients. Ketamine causes minimal loss of protective airway reflexes except in severely ill patients. If the patient is to be intubated and suxamethonium given, this benefit is lost. Intramuscular ketamine should be considered as an alternative to inhalational agents for induction in 'veinless' patients.

Essential premedication

(1) Lorazepam 2–4 mg orally or IM 1 hour preoperatively.
(2) Atropine 0.6 mg IM 1 hour preoperatively.

Dosage

Give 1–2 mg/kg IV over 60 seconds, or 4–10 mg/kg IM. Increase the dose for alcoholics.

Complications

(1) Salivation: this is reduced by atropine premedication.
(2) Emergence hallucinations: these are reduced by lorazepam premedication and allowing the patient to recover in a quiet room with minimal disturbance.
(3) Airway obstruction: this is abolished by use of an airway.
(4) Vomiting.

Suxamethonium

Indication

To provide rapid relaxation for intubation.

Absolute contraindications

(1) History of malignant hyperpyrexia.
(2) Serum potassium greater than 5.5 mmol/l.
(3) Penetrating eye injury.
(4) Myasthenia gravis.
(5) Myotonia.
(6) Paraplegia or quadriplegia associated with active muscle wasting.

(7) Massive muscle trauma.
(8) Burns in the period 1 week to 2 months after the burn.
(9) Renal failure with untreated hyperkalaemia.

Relative contraindications

(1) Liver disease.
(2) Plasma cholinesterase deficiency.

The use of suxamethonium may be considered essential even though it is relatively contraindicated. If the patient fails to breathe, postoperative ventilation is indicated.

Essential premedication

Atropine 0.6 mg IV should be administered with the first dose of suxamethonium if repeated doses of suxamethonium are to be given.

Dosage

Give 1–2 mg/kg IV. In an emergency, if a vein is not available, suxamethonium may be injected into the tongue, from where it is rapidly absorbed.

Complications

(1) Bradycardia; this follows repeated doses of suxamethonium unless atropine is given.
(2) Dysrhythmias and cardiac arrest: these may be prevented by atropine premedication.
(3) Increased intraocular pressure. Tubocurarine 3 mg IV given 3 minutes before the suxamethonium or acetazolamide 500 mg IV immediately before induction are said to prevent the increase but not everyone agrees.
(4) Bronchospasm.
(5) Increased serum potassium. This is the reason why it is contraindicated in certain cases (see pp. 66–67, items 2, 6, 7, 8 and 9).
(6) Increased intracranial pressure. The increase is transient, and its risks should be balanced against suxamethonium's other advantages.

Methods of intubation under local or general anaesthesia

The method chosen and the type of anaesthesia will depend on the problems which are likely to arise. Sometimes it will be necessary to try more than one method on the same patient.

Oral under direct vision

Indications

This is the standard method of intubation and is used when the larynx is visible on direct laryngoscopy and there are no contraindications.

Contraindications

(1) Dental or maxillofacial surgery when a tube in the mouth might get in the surgeon's way.
(2) Inability to open the mouth.

Methods

(1) Standard intubation using a laryngoscope to facilitate place-ment of the tube in the trachea. The patient's head should be placed in the 'sniffing the air' position. The curve of the tube may be increased, if necessary, by using a wire stylet. If the tube passes a small distance through the larynx and then impinges on the trachea, try rotating the tube through 90–180°. It will then usually pass easily into the trachea. Return it to its normal position before fixing. If rotating the tube does not result in tracheal intubation, try a smaller sized tube.
(2) If only the tip of the epiglottis is visible, try intubating the trachea with a long gum-elastic bougie which can be used to lift the epiglottis. The bougie can then be advanced along the inferior border of the epiglottis into the larynx and trachea. Lubricate the inside of the tube with water-soluble jelly and railroad it over the bougie into the trachea.
(3) Occasionally the larynx may be seen more easily with a rigid intubating bronchoscope. Lubricate the inside of a tube with water-soluble jelly and thread it onto the bronchoscope. Open the patient's mouth using the left hand by placing the

thumb on the upper gum or teeth and the first finger on the lower gum. Pass the bronchoscope into the mouth in the midline, supporting it on the thumb, and visualize the uvula. Extend the patient's head and pass the bronchoscope anteriorly until the larynx is seen. Intubate the trachea with the bronchoscope and then railroad the tube into the trachea.

Blind oral

Indications

These methods should not be used as the first choice. They may, however, be useful when oral intubation under direct vision has failed.

Methods

(1) Stand facing the patient and place the first and middle fingers of the left hand over the patient's tongue until the epiglottis can be felt. Pull the tongue anteriorly and guide the tube between the fingers into the larynx.

(2) Clean the neck with a suitable solution (see Appendix 2). Scrub up and wear sterile gloves; this step may be omitted if the procedure has not been planned and time is short. Choose a CVP catheter at least 80 cm long which can be introduced through a needle. Palpate the cricothyroid membrane and puncture it in the midline with a needle. Check that air can be freely aspirated. Thread the cannula through the needle in the direction of the larynx. When it has passed into the mouth, retrieve it with Magill forceps. Remove the needle and railroad the tube over the catheter into the trachea. Cut the catheter off flush with the skin and withdraw the remainder through the mouth. A Drum cartridge catheter may be used in a similar way, but there is a risk that the catheter will be threaded into the tissues as there is no way to check the position of the needle. A Tuohy needle and epidural catheter can also be used.

Nasal under direct vision

Indications

Method 1 is indicated for dental and maxillofacial surgery. Method 2 may be used as an alternative to blind nasal intubation.

Contraindications

(1) History of profuse nose bleeds.
(2) Bleeding diatheses.
(3) Anticoagulant therapy.

Methods

(1) Smear the nasal cavity with 10% cocaine paste to reduce bleeding. Lubricate a cuffed nasal tube (size 8.5 mm OD for males and 7.5 mm OD for females) with water-soluble jelly. Aspirate air from the cuff and clip the pilot tube. Pass the tube gently through whichever nostril allows its easiest passage (this is usually the side the patient finds it easiest to breathe through). Never use excessive force. Pass the tube into the oropharynx. Use a laryngoscope to visualize the larynx, and flex the patient's head so that the tube passes into the trachea. Sometimes the tube may have to be guided into the trachea with Magill forceps. Inflate the cuff, suck clot and mucus out of the tube and ventilate the lungs. A damp throat pack should be used to prevent blood clot collecting above the cuff. The size of the throat pack will depend on the site of the operation but should be as large as possible.
(2) Lubricate the inside of a cuffed nasal tube and thread it onto a fibreoptic bronchoscope. The technique is the same as for method 1, above, except that the bronchoscope is used to visualize the larynx and guide the tube into the trachea. Once the trachea is intubated, the bronchoscope is withdrawn.
   NB. This technique is difficult and should not be tried for the first time in an emergency.

Blind nasal

Indications

(1) Inability to open the mouth.
(2) Inability to visualize the epiglottis or cords.
(3) Failure of other methods.

Contraindications

(1) History of profuse nose bleeds.
(2) Bleeding diatheses.
(3) Anticoagulant therapy.

Method

Smear the nasal cavity with 10% cocaine paste. Lubricate the tube with water-soluble jelly and deflate its cuff. Advance the tube into the oropharynx. Ask the patient to take slow deep breaths if he is awake. If he is already anaesthetized and breathing oxygen, nitrous oxide and halothane, add 5% carbon dioxide to the inspired mixture. It is vital to maintain a clear airway if this technique is used. In the presence of halothane, any further increase in $PaCO_2$ may cause dysrhythmias. Place the patient's head in such a position that the anticipated path of the tube matches its curve. Listening to the breath sounds, advance the tube gently until it enters the trachea.

If the breath sounds stop or start to gurgle, the tube is in the oesophagus: withdraw the tube until normal breath sounds are heard; extend the head slightly and advance the tube again. If the tube becomes stuck when it is only two-thirds of the way in, it may be stuck in the anterior commissure: withdraw the tube and flex the head slightly; it should then pass into the trachea. It could also be stuck in the pyriform fossa, when a bulge in the neck will be seen lateral to and slightly above the larynx: withdraw the tube and rotate it medially; it should then pass into the trachea.

Having intubated the trachea, inflate the cuff and aspirate blood and mucus from the tube. Proceed with the anaesthetic.

Tracheostomy under local anaesthesia

Indications

(1) If repeated operations are planned and intubation will be difficult every time.
(2) If failure of other methods seems likely. You should consult your senior colleagues before making the final decision.
(3) Failure of other methods.

Contraindications

(1) Technical impossibility.
(2) If other techniques are likely to succeed.

Method

Tracheostomy should be performed by a surgeon who has the necessary expertise.

Using a Robertshaw tube

Indications

(1) To isolate one lung.
(2) In order to collapse one lung to improve surgical access.

Method

(1) Choose a suitable sized tube:
   small Robertshaw   ≡ 8.0 mm OD endotracheal tube
   medium Robertshaw ≡ 9.5 mm OD endotracheal tube
   large Robertshaw   ≡ 11.0 mm OD endotracheal tube
(2) Choose a left- or right-sided tube. Left-sided tubes are used for all cases except when the left main bronchus may be involved in the operation.
(3) Induce local or general anaesthesia as indicated.
(4) With the tip concavity anteriorly, insert the tip of the tube through the cords.
(5) Rotate the tube through 90° so that the shaft concavity is anterior. Advance the tube into the trachea and bronchus.
(6) Clamp the tracheal side and inflate the bronchial cuff. Check that the lung on the correct side is being ventilated. If a right-sided tube is being used, check particularly that the right upper lobe is being ventilated. This may require a slight alteration in the position of the tube. Rarely, the tube will pass down the wrong bronchus and will require resiting.
(7) Remove the tracheal clamp and inflate the tracheal cuff. Check that both lungs are equally ventilated.
(8) Fix the tube firmly and recheck its position.
(9) When the patient has been positioned on the table, check that the tube is still correctly placed.
(10) When you wish to deflate a lung, clamp either the bronchial or the tracheal side and remove the bung. Ventilate the patient with at least 50% oxygen. Check that the patient is being adequately ventilated by measuring the arterial blood gases. Avoid excessive inflation pressures by decreasing the tidal volume and increasing the rate of ventilation. Hypoxia may be minimized by insufflating oxygen at a rate of 3 litres per minute into the collapsed lung.

Establishing access to a vein

If possible, this should be done before the induction of anaesthesia. Skin infiltration with 1% lignocaine reduces the pain from insertion of a large-bore cannula.

Choosing a site

The following factors influence the siting of cannulae:

(1) Use the non-dominant arm for patient comfort.
(2) Avoid crossing joints.
(3) Insertion at the confluence of two veins is often easier.
(4) The injection port should be accessible to the anaesthetist during the operation. If this is impossible, an extension and three-way tap may be used. Always remember to flush drugs through the extension set into the vein.
(5) Cannulation of lower limb veins is often complicated by phlebitis and is best avoided if there are veins available in the arm or hand.
(6) Varicose veins should never be used.
(7) If difficulty is anticipated, start with the most distal veins because holes proximal to the site of an infusion may leak badly.

Method

(1) Apply a tourniquet at a pressure mid-way between systolic and diastolic BP, and place the limb below the level of the heart.
(2) Encourage veins to appear by tapping the skin over the site of the vein, asking the patient to repeatedly open and close his hand; if the patient is cold, place the limb in a bowl of warm water, having first tested the temperature with your *own* hand. If the limb is oedematous, press firmly over the site of a vein to disperse the oedema.
(3) Clean the skin with a suitable solution (see Appendix 2). Allow the skin to dry.
(4) If a large cannula is to be used, raise a skin bleb with 1% lignocaine a few millimetres away from the vein.
(5) Stretch the skin tautly over the vein.
(6) Insert the cannula through the bleb into the vein, watching for the blood to flash-back.

(7) Slide the cannula off the stylet into the vein. Never reinsert the stylet after it has been withdrawn.

(8) If blood fails to flow freely through the cannula, withdraw it until blood flows freely. Try to advance the cannula into the vein.

(9) Having failed to cannulate a vein, press firmly over the puncture site until the bleeding stops. Start again at a new site.

(10) Having cannulated the vein, do not forget to remove the tourniquet before connecting an infusion or injecting drugs.

Failure to cannulate a vein

Several courses of action are available:

(1) Proceed with an inhalational induction. Halothane may dilatate peripheral veins, which can be cannulated after intubation.

(2) Cut down onto a vein.

(3) Cannulate a central vein.

(4) Induce anaesthesia with IM ketamine and allow the patient to breathe oxygen and 1% halothane, which may dilatate peripheral veins.

Intubation in the awake unanaesthetized patient

Intubation without any form of anaesthetic following preoxygenation for 3 minutes is preferable for patients with obtunded reflexes. As the tube enters the trachea the patient may manage a weak cough. This method is therefore contraindicated in patients with raised intracranial pressure or penetrating eye injuries.

Intubation under local anaesthesia in the awake patient

Indications

(1) Upper respiratory tract obstruction.

(2) Difficult intubation in a patient whose airway is insecure.

(3) Hypovolaemia, dehydration, cardiac disease, etc., where there is a grave risk of hypotension with intravenous induction agents.

(4) Patients for whom an intravenous or inhalation induction could prove hazardous or is contraindicated.

Contraindications

(1) If protective airway reflexes are obtunded and intubation without anaesthesia is possible.
(2) Trauma to the oral mucosa.
(3) Lack of patient co-operation to an extent that renders the technique hazardous or technically impossible.

Premedication

(1) Droperidol 2.5–5 mg plus fentanyl 0.05–0.1 mg IM 45 minutes preoperatively, provided there is no risk of respiratory depression or obstruction.
(2) Atropine 0.6 mg IM 1 hour preoperatively to prevent salivation.

Technique of anaesthesia

See pp. 59–60.

Method of intubation

Preoxygenate the patient for 3 minutes. Then proceed as for intubation under local or general anaesthesia (pp. 68–72).

Preparation of equipment

All equipment should be prepared and checked prior to the induction of anaesthesia.

Oxygen supply

There should be a full reserve cylinder on every anaesthetic machine. The main supply may come from a cylinder or a pipeline.

(1) *Checking for correct connection of cylinders.* Switch off the cylinders and (if applicable) disconnect the pipelines from the wall, *not* from the anaesthetic machine. Open the oxygen

and nitrous oxide rotameters. Open the oxygen cylinder and check that the oxygen rotameter rises. Note also how full the cylinders are by reading the pressure gauge. Switch off the cylinder.

(2) *Checking for correct connection of the pipeline.* The procedure is similar to that for checking cylinders. When the oxygen pipeline is connected, the oxygen rotameter should rise. Disconnect the pipeline.

(3) *Checking the oxygen failure warning device.* Make sure the device is switched on. With the oxygen supply switched on and the oxygen rotameter open, disconnect the oxygen supply. The warning device should sound.

NB. Some devices function only if nitrous oxide is flowing.

These procedures ensure that gas is flowing to the correct rotameter but do not confirm that the cylinder or pipeline are actually supplying oxygen. Use of an oxygen analyser will confirm that the gas is oxygen.

Nitrous oxide supply

This may come from a cylinder or a pipeline. Use the same technique as that described for oxygen to check that connections are correct. Apart from weighing the cylinder, there is no way of checking how much nitrous oxide a cylinder contains. If a cylinder is being used, always watch the pressure dial and rotameter with great care. The pressure will fall sharply only when the cylinder is almost empty; at this time ice may be seen around the base of the cylinder.

Primary source

Before starting an anaesthetic check that reserve cylinders of oxygen and nitrous oxide are switched off and that the primary source of both gases is open.

Vaporizers

Decide which vapour you will be using and fill the appropriate vaporizer. Do not switch on the vaporizer until the vapour is needed. Check that any other vaporizers are switched off.

Anaesthetic circuits

Connect the parts together in the correct order to ensure that the connections are compatible.

(1) Circuits for spontaneous respiration consist of an anaesthetic machine, a 2 litre reservoir bag, elephant tubing of adequate length, an expiratory valve, a catheter mount and an endotracheal tube (or curved connector and face mask). Check for leaks by supplying oxygen at 1 litre per minute, turning on the vaporizer, closing the expiratory valve and occluding the end of the circuit. Leaks are indicated by a hissing noise, bubbling from the vaporizer filling port or failure of the reservoir bag to fill.

(2) Circuits for IPPV consist of hoses connected to the inspiratory and expiratory ports of the ventilator. These hoses are attached near the patient to a Y-connector which should fit the catheter mount. A reservoir bag and expiratory valve should be available on the ventilator for manual ventilation. Ventilators capable of entraining air also have a reservoir bag for anaesthetic gases. Check the circuit for leaks in the same way as for a spontaneous respiration circuit. If the ventilator has a pressure gauge, occlusion of the circuit should produce the pressure which is the maximum permitted before the relief valve operates. Low pressure indicates a leak and a high pressure indicates a faulty pressure relief valve.

Ventilator

The number of different ventilators available restricts the following comments to generalities. You should always use a ventilator with which you are familiar.

(1) Check that the ventilator is connected to the gas supply.
(2) If the gas is supplied via an anaesthetic machine, check that the correct circuit and outlet are being used.
(3) Some ventilators are electrically driven. Check that the mains and ventilator are switched on.

Set the controls:

(1) *Tidal volume:* 10 ml/kg is a common choice.
(2) *Rate:* 10–12 breaths per minute. Ventilators which have a

rate control entrain air if the anaesthetic gas supply is inadequate. Always check that the reservoir bag contains anaesthetic gases and does not collapse completely with each breath.

(3) *Minute volume.* Ventilators which are minute volume dividers should have the chosen minute volume delivered from the rotameters.

Cuffed endotracheal tubes

(1) Prepare three tubes for each patient: sizes 7.5 mm OD, 8.0 mm OD and 8.5 mm OD for females and 8.5 mm OD, 9.0 mm OD and 9.5 mm OD for males. The middle sizes are suitable for most patients. Occasionally the tubes which have been prepared are inappropriate. Tubes of other sizes should be readily available. For nasal intubation a range of tube sizes should also be prepared. The middle size should be 7.5 mm OD for females and 8.5 mm OD for males.

(2) Several types of tube are available. Red rubber tubes are used for most cases. If postoperative ventilation is planned, a non-irritant tube (e.g. Portex, Shiley) should be used. Non-kinking armoured tubes are required for head and neck operations or if the lateral or prone position is to be used.

(3) The tubes should be cut to the correct length. This is most easily done by measuring the tube against the patient.

(4) Check the cuff for leaks or asymmetry, and discard if either is present.

Connectors

These should fit tightly in the tube and be so positioned that the tube will not kink when the anaesthetic circuit is connected.

Catheter mount

The mount should fit the connector snugly and also the rest of the anaesthetic circuit.

20 ml syringe

Withdraw the plunger ready to inflate the cuff.

Clip

Clip to prevent deflation of the cuff.

Bandage or adhesive tape

This is required to fix the tube; use a method which will not encroach on the operating field.

Two laryngoscopes

Check that the correct size and variety of blade is securely attached. The light bulb should be tightened, and, if the light is dim, new batteries fitted. The second laryngoscope acts as a spare. You may wish to attach a different blade to assist with a difficult intubation.

Introducers

These should be prepared in anticipation of a difficult intubation.

(1) Wire stylet: this may be essential for the insertion of an armoured tube.
(2) Gum-elastic bougie.

Airways

Prepare sizes 2, 3 and 4, which will be suitable for most patients.

Face mask

Choose a mask which fits the patient. If the facial contour is distorted, cotton wool padding may be helpful to ensure a good fit.

Monitoring equipment

See Chapter 3.

Suction apparatus

Check that the apparatus is working and is attached to suction tubing and a suction catheter. Switch the machine on and place the suction catheter so that it may be quickly picked up if the patient vomits.

Drugs

Having first checked the contents of the ampoules, all induction agents should be drawn up in labelled syringes. (See also pp. 62–67.)

Intravenous cannula

(1) A 2 mm OD plastic cannula is essential for all patients who may need rapid transfusion of blood or clear fluid, and is advisable for all cases requiring intravenous fluids.
(2) A 1 mm OD plastic cannula or butterfly needle should be used for the induction and administration of other drugs for all patients not requiring intravenous fluids.

Intravenous fluid and drip set

Include a warming coil and filter if blood is likely to be given. If the injection port of the intravenous catheter will be inaccessible, include a three-way tap and extension set.

Tipping operating table

This is essential for the induction and recovery periods, when the patient may vomit. If a trolley is used, this too should have the facility for tipping.

Resuscitation equipment

Drugs (see pp. 127–132) and a defibrillator should be readily available.

Special equipment

This may include:

(1) Blood warmer.
(2) Warming blanket.
(3) Body supports for non-supine operating positions.

(4) Tourniquet.
(5) Throat pack.

Checking the patient

(1) Ask the patient his name and address; his answer should correspond with the notes.
(2) Check that the name and number on the patient's identity band correspond with his notes and consent form.
(3) Check that the consent form is signed and that the nature and site of the operation are correct.
(4) Check the time that the patient last ate and drank.
(5) If premedication was ordered, check that it has been given.
(6) Check that blood has been cross-matched.
(7) Check that nail varnish and lipstick, which may obscure cyanosis, have been removed.

Crash induction: intravenous induction and intubation

Indications (non-emergencies included)

(1) Milky drink, alcoholic drink or food 6 hours or more previously, depending on other factors which delay stomach emptying.
(2) Other drinks (excluding sips of water with premedication) 4 hours previously.
(3) Active or recent bleeding from the oesophagus, stomach or duodenum.
(4) Abdominal swelling due to any cause.
(5) History of hiatus hernia or oesophageal reflux.

Assumptions before use

(1) Control of the airway is assured at all times.
(2) Local anaesthetic techniques are unsuitable or contraindicated.
(3) Awake intubation without local anaesthesia is impossible.
(4) Tracheostomy under local anaesthesia is not indicated.
(5) Intravenous induction agents are not contraindicated.
(6) Surgery cannot be postponed.

Method

(1) Preoxygenation: the patient breathes 100% oxygen for 3 minutes prior to induction. To avoid dilution with air, check that the face mask fits the patient's face well. Preoxygenation creates a reservoir of oxygen in the lungs which allows induction and most intubations to be completed without ventilating the lungs or rendering the patient hypoxic until the airway is protected. Ventilation with a face mask blows gas into the stomach and increases the risk of regurgitation.

(2) The position of the patient is a matter of individual choice.
(a) A 45° head-up tilt prevents regurgitation but not vomiting. If vomiting occurs, aspiration is almost inevitable. The position aggravates hypotension from other causes.
(b) A 15° head-down tilt allows small volumes of stomach contents to drain into the pharynx where they may be sucked out. However, large volumes may still flood into the larynx. This position increases the pressure in the stomach and hence the risk of regurgitation.
(c) The supine position reduces the risks mentioned in (a) and (b). If regurgitation or vomiting occurs, the patient must be turned into the lateral position and tipped head down.

(3) Apply cricoid pressure. An assistant is *always* required to perform this task. The cricoid cartilage is pressed firmly against the vertebral column, using the thumb and first two fingers. Cricoid pressure prevents regurgitation and should not be stopped until the anaesthetist is satisfied that the lungs are protected. It should only be stopped prior to inflation of the cuff if vomiting occurs. Increased oesophageal pressure due to vomiting may rupture the oesophagus.

(4) Inject a predetermined dose of induction agent as rapidly as is consistent with the patient's cardiovascular status.

(5) In relatively fit patients, inject suxamethonium when the lid reflex is lost. In patients with a slow circulation time, wait 15 seconds and inject suxamethonium rapidly.

(6) Do *not* ventilate the patient.

(7) When the jaw relaxes, insert the laryngoscope and intubate. There is no point trying to intubate before the patient is relaxed because the patient will probably cough. Coughing induces vomiting.

(8) Inflate the cuff slowly while ventilating the patient with 100%

oxygen until the sound of leaking gas stops and the tracheobronchial tree is isolated.
 (9) Check that both lungs are being ventilated equally. This is best done by auscultation.
(10) Release cricoid pressure.
(11) Fix the tube.
(12) Proceed with the anaesthetic.

Alternative method for crash induction

Indication

This method should only be used by experienced anaesthetists for patients in whom suxamethonium is contraindicated and intubation is certain to be easy.

Method

(1) Preoxygenate the patient for 3 minutes.
(2) Apply cricoid pressure.
(3) Induce anaesthesia with pancuronium 0.1 mg/kg IV followed immediately by a predetermined dose of intravenous induction agent.
(4) When the jaw relaxes (usually after 1 minute), intubate the patient.

Inhalational induction and intubation

Indications

(1) Patients with airway problems where inhibition of spontaneous respiration might render oxygenation completely impossible.
(2) Intravenous induction agents are contraindicated.
(3) Suxamethonium is contraindicated.
(4) Following failure to cannulate a vein.

Contraindications

(1) Operations for which local anaesthesia is suitable.
(2) Patients in whom awake intubation with or without local anaesthetic is possible.

Relative contraindications

(1) Young fit patients.
(2) Patients with lung disease.
(3) Grossly obese patients.

All these patients are prone to a prolonged and stormy induction.

Method

(1) Allow the longest starvation time possible.
(2) Explain the procedure to the patient and talk to him until he is asleep, using reassuring phrases that do not require an answer.
(3) Lie the patient supine with his head in the 'sniffing the air' position.
(4) There is a choice of agents:
    (a) oxygen in 70% nitrous oxide is often enough for ill and frail patients;
    (b) oxygen in 70% nitrous oxide with up to 5% halothane;
    (c) oxygen in 70% nitrous oxide with up to 5% enflurane.
       Use lower concentrations of the volatile agent in frail or hypovolaemic patients.
(5) Place the face mask so that it fits the patient's face tightly. If the patient wishes to do so, he should be allowed to hold the mask himself.
(6) Supply oxygen and nitrous oxide through the mask. If halothane or enflurane is being given, allow the patient to take about five breaths at each concentration, starting at 0.5% and increasing in 0.5–1% increments until the maximum concentration is reached.
(7) As the lid reflex is lost, ask an assistant to apply cricoid pressure. You should support the jaw from now on.
(8) Always avoid respiratory obstruction which may induce vomiting. An airway may help provided it does not induce vomiting.
(9) During the excitement phase hold the mask firmly on the face and, if necessary, ask assistants to restrain the patient.
(10) When the patient is deeply asleep and the jaw is completely relaxed, gently insert the laryngoscope. If the cords are clearly visible and open, rapidly intubate the patient and inflate the cuff. The patient may cough if the cough reflex is still present. You may find it helpful to spray the oral cavity

and larynx with 4% lignocaine. However, if this is done too soon, coughing may be induced.

(11) When the tracheobronchial tree has been isolated, stop cricoid pressure.

Inhalational agents for maintenance of anaesthesia

Nitrous oxide

Indication

Nitrous oxide, as the sole maintenance agent, is suitable only for very frail, elderly patients. In most cases it should be supplemented with an analgesic agent or another inhalational agent.

Absolute contraindications

(1) Pneumothorax without a functioning chest drain.
(2) Lung or kidney cysts.
(3) Pneumopericardium.
(4) Recent pneumoencephalogram.
(5) Bronchial fistula without a functioning chest drain.

Relative contraindications

(1) Bowel obstruction.
(2) Eustachian tube obstruction.

Dosage

Because 30% oxygen should be given to all patients, the maximum concentration of nitrous oxide is 70%.

Complications

(1) Nausea and vomiting if anaesthesia is associated with hypoxia.
(2) Diffusion hypoxia. This is brief and may be overcome by giving 100% oxygen for 5–10 minutes after the nitrous oxide has been switched off.

Halothane

Indication

As a supplement to nitrous oxide.

Absolute contraindications

(1) Unexplained fever, jaundice or abnormal liver function tests after a previous halothane anaesthetic.
(2) Halothane anaesthetic in the previous 3 months.
(3) History of malignant hyperpyrexia.
(4) Hypercarbia.

Relative contraindications

(1) Beta-blockers.
(2) Raised intracranial pressure; 0.5% halothane may only be given to patients with raised intracranial pressure *after* they have been hyperventilated and the $PaCO_2$ reduced to approximately 3.5 kPa.
(3) Concomitant use of adrenaline. Adrenaline should be avoided if possible. If its use with halothane is unavoidable, make sure that the patient's $PaCO_2$ is normal or reduced, the maximum concentration of adrenaline is 1:400000 and the maximum dose by whatever route is not more than 100 µg per 10 minutes and 300 µg per hour. The surgeon should be actively discouraged from using adrenaline. Felypressin 1:60 (v/v) in lignocaine produces equivalent vasoconstriction. If the surgeon insists on using adrenaline, you should modify your technique and avoid the use of halothane.
(4) Patients with cardiovascular instability.
(5) Pregnancy. Concentrations greater than 0.5% cause uterine relaxation. This may cause bleeding after caesarian section. For external version, uterine relaxation is beneficial.

Dosage

(1) Spontaneous respiration: 0.5–2.5%.
(2) IPPV: 0.25–1%. Higher doses may be used briefly. Monitor the BP and decrease the dose if hypotension occurs.

Complications

(1) Bradycardia and nodal rhythm.
(2) Hypotension.
(3) Ventricular dysrhythmias.
(4) Potentiates non-depolarizing muscle relaxants. This may be turned to the anaesthetist's advantage.
(5) Decreased uterine tone.
(6) Postoperative shivering.
(7) Abnormal liver function tests, jaundice or, rarely, massive hepatic necrosis.
(8) Respiratory depression.
(9) Increased intracranial pressure.

Trichloroethylene

Indication

As a supplement to nitrous oxide when halothane is contraindicated, especially in obstetrics.

Absolute contraindication

When a soda-lime absorber is included in the anaesthetic circuit.

Relative contraindications

(1) Concomitant use of adrenaline. Follow the same procedure as for halothane (see p. 86).
(2) Beta-blockers.
(3) Anaesthesia using spontaneous respiration. Dysrhythmias are common and recovery may be prolonged.
(4) Patients with cardiovascular instability.
(5) Raised intracranial pressure. Trichloroethylene should be used only after the patient has been hyperventilated and the $Paco_2$ reduced to 3.5 kPa.

Dosage

IPPV: 0.2–0.5%.

Complications

(1) Delayed return of consciousness.
(2) Vomiting.
(3) Ventricular dysrhythmias, especially with hypercarbia.
(4) Increased intracranial pressure.

Enflurane

Indication

As a supplement to nitrous oxide when halothane is contraindicated.

Absolute contraindications

(1) Renal disease.
(2) Epilepsy.
(3) Pregnancy.
(4) Raised intracranial pressure.

Relative contraindications

(1) Beta-blockers.
(2) Concomitant use of adrenaline. Follow the same procedure as for halothane (see p. 86).
(3) Patients with cardiovascular instability.

Dosage

(1) Spontaneous respiration: 0.5–3%.
(2) IPPV: 0.5–1.5%. Monitor the BP and reduce the concentration if hypotension occurs.

Complications

(1) Hypotension.
(2) Decreases tidal volume in spontaneously breathing patients.
(3) Renal damage in patients with impaired renal function.
(4) Potentiates non-depolarizing muscle relaxants. This may be turned to the anaesthetist's advantage.
(5) Uterine relaxation.
(6) Increased intracranial pressure.

Analgesics for maintenance of anaesthesia

Fentanyl

Indications

As a supplement to nitrous oxide anaesthesia. It does not cause hypotension and is useful for patients with cardiovascular instability.

Contraindications

(1) MAOI therapy.
(2) Liver failure.
(3) Obstetric anaesthesia immediately prior to delivery of the baby.
(4) Head injury.

Relative contraindication

Patients prone to postoperative respiratory depression.

Dosage

(1) Spontaneous respiration: 0.05–0.2 mg IV given over 10 minutes lasts approximately 1 hour.
(2) IPPV: 0.2–0.5 mg IV at the beginning of an operation provides analgesia for 30–60 minutes. Give 0.05 mg increments when indicated. A dose of 50 µg/kg IV provides sufficient analgesia for operations lasting for 4–6 hours. Doses should be reduced for elderly, ill or myxoedematous patients.

Complications

(1) Respiratory depression (may occur several hours after recovery from anaesthesia).
(2) Muscular rigidity.
(3) Transient hypotension.
(4) Bradycardia.

The incidence of these complications is reduced by giving each dose slowly over 10 minutes.

Phenoperidine

Indications

(1) As a supplement to nitrous oxide anaesthesia for ventilated patients whose operation will last at least 2 hours.
(2) Suitable for patients with cardiovascular instability.

Contraindications

(1) MAOI therapy.
(2) Liver failure.
(3) Obstetric anaesthesia immediately prior to delivery of the baby.
(4) Head injury.

Relative contraindication

Patients prone to postoperative respiratory depression.

Dosage

Give 2–4 mg at the beginning of anaesthesia, and 1 mg increments when indicated.

Complications

(1) Respiratory depression.
(2) Bradycardia.
(3) Hypotension (very rarely).

Muscle relaxants for maintenance of anaesthesia

NB. All patients who have received muscle relaxants must be ventilated until adequate spontaneous respiration is re-established. Never permit a patient to be paralysed without supplementary agents to produce anaesthesia.

Suxamethonium infusion

Indications

Operations lasting less than 1 hour where paralysis with only minimal relaxation of the abdominal muscles is required (e.g. gynaecological procedures, laparoscopy and bronchoscopy).

Absolute contraindications

(1) History of malignant hyperpyrexia.
(2) Serum potassium greater than 5.5 mmol/l.
(3) Penetrating eye injury.
(4) Myasthenia gravis.
(5) Myotonia.
(6) Paraplegia or quadriplegia associated with active muscle wasting.
(7) Massive muscle trauma.
(8) Burns in the period 1 week to 2 months after the burn.
(9) Renal failure with untreated hyperkalaemia.

Relative contraindications

(1) Liver disease.
(2) Plasma cholinesterase deficiency.

Premedication

Give atropine 0.6 mg IV at induction.

Dosage

(1) Intubation: 1–2 mg/kg.
(2) Maintenance: 0.1% solution of suxamethonium in physiological saline at the rate necessary to stop spontaneous efforts to breathe and movement of limbs. Usually 140–400 ml per hour is sufficient.

Complications

(1) Dual block. Unlikely if no more than 400 mg is given over 1 hour.
(2) Tachyphylaxis.
(3) Bradycardia; this follows repeated doses of suxamethonium unless atropine is given.
(4) Dysrhythmias and cardiac arrest; these may be prevented by atropine premedication.

(5) Increased intraocular pressure. Tubocurarine 3 mg IV given 3 minutes before the suxamethonium or acetazolamide 500 mg IV immediately before induction are said to prevent the increase but not everyone agrees.
(6) Bronchospasm.
(7) Increased serum potassium. This is the reason why it is contraindicated in certain cases (see pp. 66–67, items 2, 6, 7, 8 and 9).
(8) Increased intracranial pressure. The increase is transient and its risks should be balanced against suxamethonium's other advantages.

Intermittent doses of suxamethonium

Indications

Operations lasting less than 30 minutes when paralysis is required (e.g. bronchoscopy, laparoscopy).

Contraindications

Both absolute and relative contraindications are as for suxamethonium infusion, above.

Premedication

Give atropine 0.6 mg IV at induction.

Dosage

(1) Intubation: 2 mg/kg.
(2) Increments: 10 mg whenever the patient shows any sign of muscle movement.

Complications

As for suxamethonium infusion, above.

Alcuronium

Indications

Operations where muscle relaxation is required for at least 30 minutes.

Contraindications

(1) Previous adverse reaction to alcuronium.
(2) Myasthenia gravis.
(3) Myasthenic syndrome.
(4) Asthma.
(5) Malignant hyperpyrexia.
(6) Muscle weakness.
(7) Liver disease.

Dosage

(1) Initially: 10–20 mg.
(2) Increments: 5 mg when required.

Use decreased doses for patients with renal failure or if trimetaphan is used.

Complications

(1) Respiratory paralysis.
(2) Minimal hypotension.
(3) Bronchospasm.

Pancuronium

Indications

(1) Operations where muscle relaxation is required for at least 30 minutes and an increase in blood pressure would be beneficial.
(2) Asthma.
(3) Liver disease.

Contraindications

(1) Myasthenia gravis.
(2) Myasthenic syndrome.
(3) Hypertension, whatever the cause.
(4) Muscular weakness.
(5) Atrial fibrillation.

Dosage

(1) Initially: 0.1 mg/kg.
(2) Increments: 2 mg when required.

Use decreased doses for patients with renal failure or if trimetaphan is used.

Complications

(1) Respiratory paralysis.
(2) Hypertension.
(3) Tachycardia.

Tubocurarine

Indications

Operations where muscle relaxation is required for at least 30 minutes and a decrease in blood pressure would be beneficial.

Contraindications

(1) Previous adverse reaction to tubocurarine.
(2) Myasthenia gravis.
(3) Myasthenic syndrome.
(4) Muscular weakness.
(5) Asthma.
(6) Malignant hyperpyrexia.
(7) Liver disease.

Dosage

(1) Initially: 15–45 mg.
(2) Increments: 5–10 mg when required.

Decrease the dose for patients with renal failure or if trimetaphan is used.

Complications

(1) Respiratory paralysis.
(2) Hypotension.
(3) Bronchospasm.
(4) Anaphylaxis—complications (2) and (3) are very severe.

Maintenance of anaesthesia

(1) Decide whether the patient is to be ventilated or allowed to breathe spontaneously.
(2) Ensure that the patient is asleep by giving inhalational agent(s) and/or an analgesic.
(3) Provide muscle relaxation if it is required by the surgeon.

Positioning the patient on the table

The patient should be positioned to give the best surgical access with minimum insult to the patient's cardiovascular and respiratory systems. The unconscious patient is unable to protect himself from injury. It is the anaesthetist's job to protect him.

(1) Move the patient gently to prevent abrasions and skeletal or muscle injury.
(2) Remove pooled cleaning solutions rapidly.
(3) Avoid extremes of temperature.
(4) Pad areas which may touch metal and act as pathways for electrical currents.
(5) Distribute the patient's weight evenly on the table.
(6) Pad pressure areas, including the back of the head, arms, buttocks, knees, heels and shoulders.
(7) Always uncross the patient's legs and place a pad under the ankles so that the calves do not press on the table, particularly if the patient is prone to thrombosis.
(8) Tape the eyes shut to prevent corneal abrasions.
(9) Protect the following nerves:
(a) Brachial plexus:
Never adduct the humerus to more than 90°, and if it is adducted turn the head to the same side and pronate the arm.
Do not allow the arm to fall off the edge of the table.
In the prone position, do not allow the axilla to rest against the sharp edge of a table.
In the Trendelenburg position, pad the shoulders well.
(b) Radial nerve: pad the screen where it touches the upper arm.
(c) Ulnar nerve: avoid extreme flexion of the elbow, and pad the medial epicondyle where it touches the table.

(d) Common peroneal nerve: pad lithotomy poles to prevent pressure on the fibula.

(e) Saphenous nerve: pad lithotomy poles to prevent pressure on the medial tibial condyle.

(f) Sciatic nerve: prevent straight leg extension with external rotation.

(g) Pudendal nerve: pad the orthopaedic post.

(h) Optic nerve: prevent pressure on the globe from the face mask or head support.

(i) Facial nerve: prevent excessive pressure on the ascending ramus of the mandible from your hand or the mask harness.

(j) Supraorbital nerve: prevent pressure from the catheter mount or head support.

(10) Problems of commonly used positions:

   (a) Lithotomy:

   Impaired ventilation—IPPV is the best for all but the shortest procedures.

   Left ventricular failure—raise the legs slowly in susceptible patients.

   Hypotension—lower the legs slowly in susceptible patients.

   (b) Lateral:

   Obstructed airway—use a non-kinking tube.

   Corneal abrasions—tape the eyes shut.

   (c) Lateral jack-knife:

   Impaired ventilation—IPPV is necessary. Use a non-kinking tube.

   Inferior vena caval compression and hypotension may be caused by incorrect positioning.

   Corneal abrasions—tape the eyes shut.

   (d) Prone:

   Impaired ventilation—IPPV is better than spontaneous respiration; use a non-kinking tube.

   Inferior vena caval compression and hypotension. Support the chest and pelvis so that the abdomen hangs freely.

   Corneal abrasions—tape the eyes shut.

Use of tourniquets

A tourniquet will provide a bloodless operating field for surgery on a limb. Its use is absolutely contraindicated for patients with sickle cell disease, sickle cell thalassaemia and sickle cell haemoglobin C disease. Theoretically it is safe for patients with sickle cell trait if the limb is first completely exsanguinated. This is very difficult to achieve.

In susceptible patients, cardiac failure may be precipitated if tourniquets are applied to two limbs at once. Hypotension may follow simultaneous deflation of tourniquets on two limbs. It is customary to apply a tourniquet for a maximum of 2 hours; 3 hours is probably safe.

Nerve damage may occur if the tourniquet is placed near joints where the tissues are thin. Always apply the tourniquet over the mid-upper arm or mid-thigh where fat and muscle will provide protection for the nerves.

Drugs given intravenously cannot reach a limb isolated by a tourniquet. Use inhalational agents to abolish reflex movements.

Fluid replacement

Insensible loss during operation

Replace such loss with dextrose saline or Hartmann's solution, giving 2 ml/kg per hour.

Blood loss during operation

Losses less than 1 litre

Replace blood loss of less than 1 litre with physiological saline or Hartmann's solution. Because of redistribution of electrolyte solutions, it may be necessary to give up to four times the volume of blood lost.

Losses greater than 1 litre

If blood loss is likely to be greater than 1 litre, begin replacement with up to 2 litres of physiological saline or Hartmann's solution. Blood or colloidal solutions should then be used.

(1) *Whole blood.* Cross-matched, warmed and filtered blood should be given. It is usual to give 10% calcium gluconate 10 ml with every 5 units of blood, but this is probably unnecessary if each unit is transfused over at least 5 minutes. Sodium bicarbonate should be given (see p. 17) to correct the metabolic acidosis associated with massive transfusions. Old blood contains inactive platelets and decreased amounts of clotting factors. For massive transfusion, it is better to use fresh blood (less than 24 hours old). Alternatively, clotting factors and platelets may be given.

If cross-matched blood is not available, give blood of the patient's own group or O-negative blood after using colloid solutions.

(2) *Human plasma protein fraction.* When used to replace blood:

Maximum volume HPPF given = patient's blood volume

$$\times \quad \frac{(\text{Patient's haemoglobin} - 10)}{\text{Patient's haemoglobin}}$$

The patient's haemoglobin will then be approximately 10 g/dl. Most of the human plasma protein fraction remains in the circulation for 4 hours. For early blood replacement, a volume equivalent to the volume of blood lost should be transfused.

(3) *Dextran 70* in 5% dextrose or physiological saline solution. Before giving dextran 70, take blood for cross-matching. Then transfuse up to 1500 ml dextran 70 at a maximum rate of 1 ml/kg per minute to replace an equivalent volume of blood. Dextran 70 is contraindicated if the patient is allergic to it or has a bleeding diathesis. Rarely, dextran causes anaphylactoid shock.

(4) *Haemaccel* is contraindicated if there is a history of allergy to it. For losses between 1500 and 4000 ml, replace with an equivalent volume of fluid consisting of blood and Haemaccel in equal volumes. For losses greater than 4000 ml, replace with an equivalent volume of fluid consisting of 2 parts blood to 1 part Haemaccel. Haemaccel is lost from the circulation after 4 hours.

Replacement clotting factors

Following massive transfusion of old blood, clotting may be inadequate. Do a clotting screen and treat deficiencies.

(1) *Fresh frozen plasma.* Give 2 units for every 6 units of old blood.
(2) *Platelets.* Six packs will usually raise the patient's platelet count by $100 \times 10^9/l$.

Never give clotting factors until major blood vessels have been tied. The clotting factors will be lost in the spilled blood.

Plasma loss

This usually occurs with chronic disease. Replacement should be done preoperatively with human plasma protein fraction or dextran 70.

Urine output and nasogastric aspirate

Measure these outputs hourly, and replace with 5% dextrose or physiological saline solution.

Monitoring during fluid replacement

To determine the adequacy of fluid replacement, correlate the following: (1) heart rate, (2) BP, (3) CVP, (4) core/skin temperature difference and (5) urine output.

Remember that other reasons may exist for an individual abnormality. It is particularly important to monitor the CVP when dextran 70 is given. Being hyperosmolar, it draws fluid into the circulation and could, therefore, precipitate heart failure.

Non-anaesthetic drugs given by the anaesthetist

Heparin

For vascular surgery the dose is approximately 100 units/kg IV.

Protamine

Protamine 1 mg neutralizes 100 units of heparin when given within 15 minutes of the heparin. If a longer time has elapsed less will be required. It is easiest to inject 10 mg of protamine every half minute until clotting is seen in the wound or on the swabs. Always inject protamine slowly to prevent hypotension.

Dextran 70

Dextran 70 500 ml infused slowly over the course of the operation may prevent thrombosis in patients with a history of deep vein thrombosis or pulmonary embolism.

Mannitol 20%

A dose of 1.5–2 g/kg infused over 30–60 minutes will reduce intracranial pressure.

Acetazolamide

Acetazolamide 500 mg IV reduces intraocular pressure.

Antibiotics

Before giving an antibiotic, check whether or not the patient is allergic to it, remembering also possible cross-sensitivity. Note possible interactions with anaesthetic agents (see Appendix 1). Always follow the manufacturer's instructions regarding dilution and rate of administration.

Reversal of anaesthesia

Physiotherapy

Chest physiotherapy prior to extubation facilitates removal of bronchial secretions and should be considered for all patients with chest problems preoperatively.

Suction

Suction down the endotracheal tube is indicated for removal of bronchial and tracheal secretions. It is contraindicated, however, if pulmonary oedema is present.

Give the patient 100% oxygen. Under sterile conditions, pass a catheter with a diameter not greater than half the internal diameter of the tube, down the tube. Apply suction and withdraw the catheter over 3–5 seconds. Reoxygenate the patient prior to passing another catheter or before extubation. Never use the same catheter twice.

Termination of anaesthesia

Reversal of anaesthesia which does not include non-depolarizing muscle relaxants

(1) Switch off all anaesthetic gases, except oxygen, and the suxamethonium drip (if applicable).
(2) Allow the patient to breathe pure oxygen or oxygen-enriched air.
(3) Turn the patient into the lateral position.
(4) Under direct vision, suck out pharyngeal secretions.
(5) Aspirate the nasogastric tube (if applicable).
(6) When the patient coughs, extubate him.
(7) Unless contraindicated (check appropriate entry in Chapter 9), give 35% oxygen via a face mask and suck out pharyngeal secretions until the patient is fully awake.
(8) 35% oxygen via a mask should be continued for at least 4 hours for patients who are anaemic or cold and shivering. It should also be given to patients who have heart or respiratory diseases. After major surgery, all patients will benefit from oxygen.

Reversal of non-depolarizing relaxants

(1) Conditions for reversal:
(a) when 30 minutes have elapsed since the initial dose of relaxant, or muscular movement is evident.
(b) when 15 minutes have elapsed since the last incremental dose of muscle relaxant, or muscular movement is evident.
(c) Halothane, enflurane or trichloroethylene have been switched off for 10 minutes.
(2) Give neostigmine 0.07 mg/kg (maximum 5 mg) and atropine 0.02 mg/kg together IV.
(3) As soon as the patient begins to breathe spontaneously, ventilate with 100% oxygen or oxygen-enriched air.
(4) Under direct vision, suck out the pharynx.
(5) Aspirate the nasogastric tube (if applicable).

(6) Turn the patient to the lateral position.
(7) Extubate the patient when he is breathing well and the cough reflex is present. Patients with raised intracranial pressure or who have had open eye operations should be extubated when they are breathing well—if possible, before the cough reflex returns. Then proceed as described in steps 7 and 8 on p. 101.

Postoperative ventilation

Indications for postoperative ventilation include:

(1) Failure to breathe adequately at the end of the operation.
(2) Following major surgery, particularly if large doses of analgesics have been given, the patient is cold or the work of breathing would put a significant strain on the myocardium.
(3) Following a craniotomy to reduce cerebral oedema.

Postoperative intensive care

Patients who require special monitoring or nursing procedures should be sent to the intensive care unit. Specific indications will vary from hospital to hospital. If in doubt, send the patient to the intensive care unit. He can always be transferred to a ward if a more deserving patient needs the bed.

Returning the patient to the ward

Before the patient is returned to an ordinary ward (i.e. not to the intensive care unit), check that the following criteria have been met:

(1) The patient is breathing well.
(2) The pulse, blood pressure and CVP are at acceptable levels and are stable.
(3) The patient is able to maintain his own airway.
(4) The patient is responding to commands.
(5) Postoperative analgesia, fluids and oxygen have, if necessary, been prescribed.
(6) Special nursing instructions have been written and explained to the nurse collecting the patient.

Allowing the patient to go home after general anaesthesia

The following criteria must be met:

(1) Instructions should have been given preoperatively:
(a) The patient should go home by taxi or private car, and be accompanied by a relative or friend.
(b) He should stay in bed or at least rest for 24 hours.
(c) A relative or friend should be in the house to nurse him for 24 hours.
(d) Alcohol should be avoided for 24 hours.
(e) The patient must not drive or operate dangerous machinery or household equipment for 24 hours.
(f) If he is worried, he should contact his own doctor or the hospital immediately.
(2) Postoperatively the patient should be alert. He should be able to dress himself and walk unaided without difficulty.
(3) The instructions given preoperatively should have been repeated verbally and handed to the patient in written form.
(4) Mild analgesics only should be adequate for pain relief.
(5) There have been no anaesthetic complications and none is anticipated.
(6) There are no surgical reasons for admitting the patient.

Problems occurring during anaesthesia

Inability to cannulate a vein

For the action to take when unable to cannulate a vein, see p. 74.
see p. 74

Intra-arterial injection of irritant solutions

Causes

(1) Aberrant or superficial course of the artery.
(2) Failure to note the bright red colour and pulsation of the blood.

Symptoms and signs

(1) Pain, usually but not always severe and felt distal to the injection site.
(2) Blanching or discoloration of the skin distal to the injection site may occur.
(3) Absent pulse distal to the injection site sometimes occurs.
(4) Hypotension sometimes occurs.

Treatment

(1) Leave the needle *in situ* if you have not already removed it.
(2) Postpone the operation until treatment has been carried out. If the patient's life is in jeopardy, proceed with the anaesthetic and carry out further treatment while the operation is in progress. This may necessitate calling another anaesthetist to provide continuing care while you are occupied with treatment of the intra-arterial injection.

(3) Inject 0.5–1% procaine *without adrenaline* 10–20 ml or papaverine 10–40 mg in 5 ml Ringer-lactate solution into the artery.
(4) Provide a sympathetic block by doing a supraclavicular brachial plexus block (see pp. 50–51). If you know how to do a stellate ganglion block, specific sympathetic blockade can be achieved.
(5) *After* having performed a brachial plexus block, give heparin 10 000 units intra-arterially.
(6) Treat hypotension with intravenous physiological saline, human plasma protein fraction or dextran 70. If these fail, give methoxamine 10 mg IV.
(7) If respiration is inadequate, intubate and ventilate; 50% nitrous oxide with oxygen will provide analgesia until the brachial plexus block is effective.
(8) If the brachial plexus block is incomplete, consider the use of a systemic vasodilator (e.g. 1% tolazoline 50 ml IV). Use narcotic analgesics to provide additional pain relief.
(9) Elevate the arm to minimize oedema.
(10) In the long term, give heparin 10 000 units 6-hourly and repeat the brachial plexus block.

Inability to intubate when a patent airway can be maintained

Manoeuvres to assist intubation

If the patient has been adequately preoxygenated there will be a few minutes before the onset of hypoxia is imminent. Consideration of the following questions may help you to intubate the patient before ventilation becomes necessary:

(1) Is the patient positioned correctly in the 'sniffing the air' position?
(2) Is the assistant applying cricoid pressure correctly or is the trachea deviated to one side?
(3) Would a gum-elastic bougie or wire stylet facilitate intubation?
(4) Would a smaller tube pass more easily into the trachea?
(5) Was the dose of relaxant adequate?
(6) Could you use another technique for intubation?

Failed intubation

While attempting to intubate, it is important that the patient does not become hypoxic. It may be necessary to ventilate the patient before he has been intubated. To minimize the risk of aspiration, the failed intubation drill should be followed:

(1) Ask someone to call a senior anaesthetist and ask for assistance.
(2) Place the patient head down in the lateral position.
(3) Maintain the cricoid pressure.
(4) Oxygenate the patient by manually ventilating through a face mask.
(5) Decide whether it is essential to carry on with the operation immediately (e.g. caesarian section for severe fetal distress). If this is so, manually ventilate the patient with nitrous oxide and oxygen until spontaneous respiration returns.
(6) Pass a large-bore stomach tube and remove any stomach contents.
(7) Instil 30 ml magnesium trisilicate down the stomach tube.
(8) Remove the stomach tube.
(9) Suck any secretions out of the pharynx.
(10) Add a suitable volatile agent supplement to the nitrous oxide.
(11) Return the patient to the horizontal position and allow the surgeon to proceed.
(12) Cricoid pressure should be maintained until the stomach tube has been removed. It may then be released, although increased protection is obtained if cricoid pressure is maintained throughout the operation.
(13) If the operation can be delayed for a short time, ventilate the patient with 100% oxygen until spontaneous respiration is established and allow him to wake up. When your senior colleague arrives, he will decide how best to proceed.

Inability to intubate if the airway cannot be maintained

Manoeuvres to aid airway maintenance

If the airway is impossible to maintain, check the following:

(1) Is the head extended, with the jaw pushed upwards and forwards by pressure on the vertical ramus of the mandible?

(2) Does the face mask fit the face well? Would cotton wool help to fill the gaps?
(3) Would a different size airway be better?
(4) Would a stitch through the tongue enable you to pull it forward and clear the airway?

Failed intubation

If you have not secured the airway and spontaneous respiration is not returning:

(1) Pass two 2 mm OD cannulae through the cricothyroid membrane in the midline. Check that air can be aspirated through both. Connect one cannula to a supply of oxygen flowing at 8 litres per minute. Intermittently occlude the other cannula with a finger to provide IPPV.
   (a) If this too fails, an emergency tracheostomy is indicated.

Submucous passage of the endotracheal tube

(1) Observe the patient for signs of impending respiratory obstruction due to haematoma or oedema. Intubation or a tracheostomy may be required to maintain the airway.
(2) Give ampicillin 500 mg orally, four times daily for 5 days.

Torrential bleeding following nasal intubation

(1) Pack the nasal cavity with 0.5 inch (approx. 1 cm) ribbon gauze soaked in adrenaline.
(2) If bleeding comes from the post-nasal space, pass a 12 gauge Foley catheter down each nostril into the pharynx. Under direct vision, inflate each balloon with 5–10 ml air.
(3) Pull the Foley catheters so that the balloons impact in the post-nasal space. If the balloons are inflated correctly they will be just visible in front of the soft palate.
(4) Secure the position of the balloons by tying the catheters together with tape as they emerge from the nostrils.
(5) Do not cut the Foley catheters—this will cause deflation of the balloons.

Inhalation of gastric contents

(1) Place the patient head down in the lateral position and suck out the pharynx.

(2) Intubate the patient and inflate the cuff as quickly as possible.

(3) Check the pulse. Reflex cardiac arrest may have occurred; see pp. 127–132 for treatment.

(4) If the patient has not yet become cyanosed, pass a suction catheter down the tube before ventilating him with 100% oxygen. Continue to suck out the trachea and ventilate the patient alternately until no further aspirate is obtained. Check the pH of the aspirate, as this will correlate well with mortality and morbidity.

(5) If solid or semi-solid gastric contents have been aspirated, urgent bronchoscopy is indicated.

(6) Bronchial lavage is contraindicated.

(7) Give methylprednisolone 30 mg/kg IV. Continue postoperatively, giving 30 mg/kg 8-hourly for a maximum of 48 hours.

(8) Antibiotics should be withheld until an organism has been cultured.

(9) Ventilate the patient and maintain the PaO_2 between 8 and 13.3 kPa using oxygen up to 50% and the lowest level of positive end-expiratory pressure (PEEP) compatible with an adequate PaO_2. Cancel the operation if possible until the aspiration has been fully treated. If this is not possible and a high inspired oxygen concentration is necessary, provide anaesthesia with an Althesin infusion (see p. 64). Continue to ventilate the patient postoperatively.

(10) Correct hypovolaemia (which may occur in the presence of a normal CVP) with human plasma protein fraction or whole blood if the haematocrit is less than 30%. It is best to administer these fluids in 200 ml aliquots, noting the effect of each aliquot on the CVP.

(11) If the base deficit is greater than 8, give sodium bicarbonate (see p. 17).

(12) Having treated hypoxia and hypovolaemia, bronchospasm should be treated with salbutamol 1–5 μg per minute IV until the bronchospasm eases or the pulse rate increases by more than 10 beats per minute (see p. 135).

(13) If the operation is mandatory, monitor the blood gases closely so that hypoxia is detected and quickly corrected. Correct continuing hypovolaemia.

Failure to relax

Tissued cannula

Check that the cannula is still in a vein. If it is not, resite it and give a further dose of relaxant.

Wrong drug

Recheck the ampoule. If the wrong drug has been given, prepare for possible side-effects. Give the correct relaxant.

Inadequate dose of relaxant

See pp. 90–94 for doses. Give more if an inadequate dose has been given.

Arteriopathic patient

In such a patient with poor peripheral circulation, provide additional relaxation with halothane or enflurane.

Tourniquet isolating a limb

Provide relaxation with halothane or enflurane.

Contractures

These will not be abolished by muscle relaxants.

Defective muscle relaxant

Check the batch number and give a dose of relaxant from a different batch.

Masseter muscle spasm

Such spasm following suxamethonium may be the first indication of malignant hyperpyrexia and is an indication for temperature monitoring. Intubation may be difficult (see pp. 105–107).

Generalized muscle spasm

This will occur if suxamethonium is given to a patient with myotonia dystrophica. Intubation may be difficult (see pp. 105–107).

Cyanosis

Causes of cyanosis include the following.

Failed oxygen supply

Check the contents of the cylinder. Check the rotameter bobbin's level and ensure that it is revolving freely. Check the anaesthetic circuit for disconnection. If there is any doubt about the oxygen supply, use your own expired air to oxygenate the patient by blowing down the tube.

Respiratory obstruction

Signs in addition to cyanosis include tracheal tug, see-saw breathing and rib recession.

(1) If this occurs while the patient is not intubated, extend the head and push the jaw upwards and forwards by pressing on the vertical ramus of the mandible.
(2) If the patient is intubated, check for obstruction or kinking of the endotracheal tube, catheter mount or circuit. This may be done by inspecting the circuit and catheter mount, and by attempting to pass a suction catheter down the endotracheal tube which may be impinging against the tracheal wall, kinked, or blocked by secretions or blood.

Endobronchial intubation

Signs include unequal chest movement, unequal air entry into the lungs and mild difficulty inflating the chest. Withdraw the tube slowly until the signs disappear.

Pneumothorax

The signs are similar to those of endobronchial intubation but do not improve when the tube is withdrawn.

(1) As emergency treatment, insert a 2 mm OD cannula through the chest wall in the second intercostal space at the mid-clavicular line on the side where diminished breath sounds are heard.

(2) Release of air is an indication for inserting a 26 French gauge chest drain in the same site as the cannula.

(3) Nitrous oxide should be discontinued immediately a pneumothorax has been diagnosed and anaesthesia provided with intravenous agents.

(4) Connect the chest drain to an underwater seal. Correct function is indicated by a freely swinging water level in the underwater tube. Bubbles should appear at the end of the tube, indicating that gas is being expelled from the chest.

(5) When the pneumothorax is being adequately treated with a chest drain, nitrous oxide may be recommenced.

Inadequate ventilation of all or part of the lungs

The most important sign is diminished air entry.

Segmental, lobar or whole lung collapse caused by clot or secretions

If hypoxia is severe, immediate bronchoscopy is indicated. Until it is performed, increase the inspired oxygen concentration. If hypoxia is not severe, increase the inspired oxygen concentration and perform bronchoscopy at the end of the operation.

Pulmonary oedema

Pink, frothy sputum aspirated from the tube is diagnostic. If the patient is breathing spontaneously, change to IPPV. Give frusemide 40 mg IV.

Bronchospasm

See p. 135.

Inadequate blood flow to the lungs

Causes include the following.

Hypotension

See pp. 124–126.

Myocardial failure

This is confirmed by an increased CVP level. Give frusemide 40 mg IV and consider giving ouabain 250–500 µg IV slowly for rapid digitalization.

Pulmonary embolism

Early diagnosis is difficult. The classic ECG pattern shows right heart strain, P pulmonale in leads II and III, prominent S waves in lead I and deep Q waves in lead III. Treat bronchospasm with aminophylline 250 mg slowly IV (see p. 135). Cardiac arrest or severe hypotension requires immediate surgical intervention. Increasing the inspired oxygen concentration will not alleviate the cyanosis.

Anaphylaxis

See p. 126.

Malignant hyperpyrexia

Other clinical features are masseter muscle spasm with sux-amethonium, unexplained rapid increase in core temperature, unexplained tachycardia and dysrhythmias, tachypnoea and, in some cases, muscle rigidity. Treatment is as follows:

(1) Hyperventilate with 50% nitrous oxide in oxygen to maintain $PaCO_2$ within normal limits. Discontinue all other inhalational agents.
(2) Give dantrolene 2–2.5 mg/kg IV stat.
(3) Treat metabolic acidosis with sodium bicarbonate (see p. 17). Up to 1000 mmol may be required.
(4) Measure serum electrolytes and sugar. Give 50% dextrose 25 g and 10 units soluble insulin IV stat. If serum potassium is greater than 7 mmol/l give also 10% calcium gluconate 5 ml IV.
(5) Restore the circulating volume with chilled physiological saline solution. Start immediately and do not wait for the first bag to be chilled.
(6) Having rehydrated the patient, induce a diuresis with frusemide 40 mg IV or 20% mannitol 50–100 g IV.

(7) Treat tachycardia or dysrhythmias with propranolol 1–2 mg IV.
(8) Cool the patient. This is best achieved by peritoneal lavage with chilled physiological saline or cardiopulmonary bypass. Surface cooling is inefficient but ice chips should be placed over the heart, axillary and femoral arteries.
(9) Cancel the operation until the malignant hyperpyrexia has been treated.

Reduced capillary filling

In the forehead

This may be due to any of the following.

Hypotension

See pp. 124–126.

Inadequate anaesthesia

Other signs include tachycardia, hypertension, sweating, muscle movement and tear formation. Check that the vaporizer is not empty, that nitrous oxide is being supplied at the correct flow rate and that the ventilator is not entraining air. If necessary, give additional anaesthetic agents.

Myocardial failure

See p. 112.

In the digits

The causes include those given for poor forehead capillary filling, but could also be due to cold.

Reduced venous filling

Causes include the following.

Hypotension

See pp. 124–126.

Hypovolaemia

Other signs include decreased urine output and decreased CVP. Increase the transfusion rate and check that you have accurately assessed fluid loss.

Inadequate anaesthesia

See p. 113.

Myocardial failure

See p. 112.

Tear formation

This, like reduced capillary filling, is due to inadequate anaesthesia (see p. 113).

Sweating

Sweating (which is abolished by atropine and hyoscine pre-medication) may indicate any of the following.

Inadequate anaesthesia

See p. 113.

Hypercarbia

This is often associated with hypertension and ventricular premature beats. Causes include the following.

Hypoventilation

If the patient is breathing spontaneously, assist ventilation or change to IPPV. If the patient is already on IPPV, check that the minute volume is adequate and increase if necessary.

Respiratory obstruction

See p. 110.

Exogenous carbon dioxide

Check that the carbon dioxide rotameter is switched off.

Dead space

Check the circuit for inadvertent insertion of dead space, causing excessive rebreathing.

Exclusion of carbon dioxide absorber

This device is always required for closed-circuit anaesthesia which utilizes low gas flows.

Intraperitoneal carbon dioxide

These patients should be hyperventilated to prevent hypercarbia.

Malignant hyperpyrexia

These patients also sweat due to increased body temperature (see pp. 112–113).

Hypoxia

Other signs include cyanosis (see pp. 110–113) and hypertension. Hypotension occurs with prolonged hypoxia.

Hypoglycaemia

This is associated with a rapid, thready pulse. Check the blood sugar with Dextrostix and, if low, give 50% dextrose 25 ml IV.

Vagal stimulation

This is often due to traction on the mesentery or oesophagus. It needs no treatment except removal of the stimulus unless associated with bradycardia or hypotension. In the presence of bradycardia or hypotension, however, give atropine 0.3–0.6 mg IV.

Increased core temperature

Causes include the following.

Excessive ambient temperature and humidity

These should be reduced.

Overuse of plastic or rubber surgical drapes

These should be removed.

Infection

Avoid using antibiotics unless an organism has been cultured and its sensitivity is known. Pyrexia due to infection is best left untreated unless the core temperature is greater than 40°C. Then use conservative measures such as reduction in ambient temperature, cold fluids, removal of unnecessary drapes and tepid sponging of exposed skin.

Malignant hyperpyrexia

See pp. 112–113.

Muscular movements

Swallowing and coughing in the spontaneously breathing patient or attempts to breathe, hiccoughs and limb or eye movements in paralysed patients indicate either that the patient is not adequately anaesthetized or that the non-depolarizing muscle relaxant is wearing off. These should be treated by increasing the concentration of halothane, enflurane or trichloroethylene, or by giving an increment of analgesic or non-depolarizing muscle relaxant. Check that the ventilator is not entraining air.

Rashes

Drug reaction

Rashes are quite common with many induction agents and tubocurarine. Sometimes the rash is associated with a more severe reaction, including bronchospasm and hypotension, which will require treatment (see pp. 135 and 124–126).

Transfusion reaction

(1) Stop the blood.
(2) Continue the infusion with physiological saline solution or a different unit of blood through a *clean* administration set.
(3) Give chlorpheniramine 10 mg IV.
(4) Treat bronchospasm with aminophylline 250 mg IV slowly.
(5) Treat hypotension with human plasma protein fraction, Haemaccel or a fresh unit of blood.
(6) Severe bronchospasm or hypotension may require adrenaline 0.2–0.5 mg SC (see p. 135).
(7) If haematuria occurs, give mannitol 12.5 g IV to promote a diuresis, and replace fluid lost with 5% dextrose solution.

Anaphylaxis

See p. 126.

Decreased bleeding from the wound

Causes include the following.

Tourniquet

Do not let a tourniquet confuse you.

Adrenaline infiltration

This should be a rare event without your prior knowledge. Check with the surgeon.

Local anaesthetic techniques

Spinal and epidural anaesthesia reduce the bleeding in some abdominal and pelvic operations.

Cardiac arrest

Diagnose this by checking the carotid pulse. For treatment, see pp. 127–132.

Hypotension

Check the BP. For treatment, see pp. 124–126.

Increased bleeding from the wound

Arterial and venous bleeding should be treated surgically. Capillary oozing may indicate any of the following.

Hypercarbia

This is only a serious problem during head and neck procedures.
  For causes and treatment, see pp. 114–115.

Hypoxia

For causes and treatment, see pp. 110–113.

Increased venous pressure

This is only a serious problem during head and neck operations. It is caused by coughing and straining at induction. During the operation check that:

(1) Venous return is not obstructed by the tape used to fix the tube.
(2) The head is not turned excessively to one side.
(3) The head is raised above the level of the heart.
(4) If IPPV is used, the pattern of ventilation gives the minimum mean intrathoracic pressure compatible with adequate oxygenation and mild hypocarbia.

Transfusion reaction

See p. 117.

Platelet deficiency

This may be secondary to massive blood transfusion or due to an undiagnosed preoperative deficiency state. Do a platelet count. If platelets are less than $50\,000 \times 10^9$/l, *either* give 6 packs of platelet concentrate *or* continue the blood transfusion with fresh whole blood (i.e. less than 24 hours old).

Clotting factor deficiency

This may be secondary to massive blood transfusion, a preoperative deficiency state or anticoagulant therapy.

(1) Confirm the diagnosis by checking the prothrombin time and partial thromboplastin time.
(2) Give 4 units of fresh-frozen plasma; *or*
(3) Continue the transfusion with fresh blood; *or*
(4) Give specific clotting factor concentrates if there is a known preoperative deficiency.

Ionized calcium deficiency

Theoretically, this could occur following massive blood transfusion. An empirical dose of 5% calcium chloride 5 ml may be given.

Increased capillary fragility

A rare condition, this is usually due to undiagnosed von Willebrand's disease. Ethamsylate 750 mg IV may help. Clotting factors may also be required for von Willebrand's disease.

Disseminated intravascular coagulation

This is usually associated with septicaemia or obstetric emergencies. Ask a haematologist to assist with diagnosis and treatment.

Fibrinolysis

Ask a haematologist to assist with diagnosis and treatment.

Aspirin therapy

A platelet infusion may help.

Tachycardia

Causes include the following.

Preoperative anxiety

This will be abolished by adequate anaesthesia. Record its presence for the benefit of future anaesthetists.

Pain

See p. 113.

Drug-induced

Agents which may cause tachycardia include pancuronium, gallamine and atropine. Treatment is usually unnecessary, although carotid sinus massage may be tried. Avoid other causes of tachycardia.

Hypercarbia

See pp. 114–115.

Hypoxia

See pp. 110–113.

Hypovolaemia

Estimate the fluid balance and measure the CVP and urine output. Replace fluids appropriately.

Hypotension

See pp. 124–126.

Transfusion reactions

See p. 117.

Increased core temperature

See p. 116.

Adrenocortical insufficiency

Give hydrocortisone 100 mg IV.

Thyrotoxicosis

Give propranolol 1–2 mg IV if the tachycardia causes hypotension.

Pulmonary embolism

See p. 112.

Phaeochromocytoma

See Chapter 9.

Metabolic acidosis

See p. 17.

Air embolism

See p. 136.

Atrial or ventricular dysrhythmias

See pp. 132–134.

Hypoglycaemia

If the blood sugar is low, give 50% dextrose 25 g IV.

Bradycardia

Drug-induced

Agents which may be responsible include suxamethonium, digitalis, halothane, analgesics and anticholinesterases. Treat with atropine 0.6 mg IV and decrease the dose of halothane. Bradycardia may also be caused by beta-blockers. Try atropine 1.2 mg IV and, if associated with hypotension, an isoprenaline infusion (see Appendix 3).

Severe hypoxia

See pp. 110–113.

Reflex autonomic response

This may be due to eyeball traction or pressure, traction on the peritoneum or anal canal, or cervical dilatation. Remove the cause; if this is not possible or ineffective, give atropine 0.6 mg IV.

Dysrhythmias or myocardial conduction defects

See pp. 132–134.

Raised intracranial pressure

See p. 138.

Hypertension

Causes include the following.

Intubation

Intubation may be a cause, especially if induction is stormy. Treat by quickly deepening the anaesthesia.

Painful stimuli

Inadequate anaesthesia

See p. 113. If it is impossible to provide adequate anaesthesia, consider infusing sodium nitroprusside or trimetaphan (see Appendix 3).

Distended bladder

Catheterize the bladder or try deepening anaesthesia. The choice made depends on which method is least harmful to the patient.

Hypercarbia

See pp. 114–115.

Hypoxia

See pp. 110–113.

Drug-induced

Pancuronium and vasopressors may be responsible for hypertension. Try reversing with halothane.

Overtransfusion

(1) Try halothane, chlorpromazine 10–50 mg IV or a sodium nitroprusside infusion (see Appendix 3).
(2) If severe, venesection may be necessary.

Raised intracranial pressure

See p. 138.

Phaeochromocytoma

See Chapter 9.

Carcinoid tumour

See Chapter 9.

Hypotension

Overdose of anaesthetic agent

Overdose may be relative.

(1) Elevate the feet.
(2) Reduce the concentration of halothane or enflurane.
(3) If the operation has not begun, encourage the surgeons to begin quickly as this is often sufficient stimulus to overcome the effects of induction agents.
(4) Rapidly infuse 1 litre physiological saline solution.
(5) If steps 1–4 fail, give ephedrine 10 mg IV. This may need to be repeated if hypotension returns.
(6) Check that sodium nitroprusside or similar infusions are switched off.

Hypovolaemia

Inadequate preoperative resuscitation

Infuse appropriate fluid (physiological saline solution, human plasma protein fraction or blood).

Incorrect assessment of blood loss

Reassess losses and correct the deficit.

Dysrhythmias

See pp. 132–134.

Myocardial failure

Give ouabain 250–500 µg IV slowly. If this fails, try a dopamine infusion (see Appendix 3).

Impeded venous return

Positional

(1) If it is essential to have the legs in a dependent position, try bandaging them.

(2) If the patient is in the lateral jack-knife position, check that supports are not occluding the inferior vena cava.
(3) In the prone position, check that the chest and pelvis are adequately raised so that the abdomen hangs freely.

Retractors

Retractors, particularly those in the region of the liver, may obstruct the inferior vena cava.

Positive end-expiratory pressure

This raises the mean intrathoracic pressure. Check the ventilator for the addition of PEEP and make sure that the expiratory valves are fully open.

Tension pneumothorax

See p. 110.

Reflex autonomic response

This may be due to eyeball traction or pressure, traction on the peritoneum or anal canal and cervical dilatation. Hypotension is associated with a bradycardia.

(1) Remove the stimulus.
(2) If this is ineffective or the stimulus is likely to recur, give atropine 0.6 mg IV.

Adrenal insufficiency

This usually occurs in patients with a history of steroid therapy. Give hydrocortisone 100–200 mg IV.

Septic shock

Septic shock usually follows manipulation of the large bowel or a large abscess. For treatment, see p. 20. If an organism has already been cultured and its sensitivity is known, use the appropriate antibiotic.

Anaphylactic shock

Anaphylactic shock may occur a few minutes after the administration of an anaesthetic drug, antibiotic, blood, dextran 70 or Haemaccel.

Signs

Signs, apart from hypotension, are:

(1) Cyanosis.
(2) Rash.
(3) Flushing or pallor.
(4) Bronchospasm.

Treatment

(1) If the anaphylactic shock is due to an infusion, stop it and change the giving set.
(2) Ventilate with 100% oxygen.
(3) Treat hypotension with physiological saline solution and human plasma protein fraction.
(4) Adrenaline 0.5 mg given slowly IV will alleviate hypotension and bronchospasm. The same dose may be given subcutaneously but impaired absorption may reduce the effect (see also p. 135).
(5) Methylprednisolone 30 mg/kg IV.

Increased CVP

Check that the measuring device is correctly zeroed before instituting treatment.

Fluid overload

(1) Check the fluid balance and withhold further fluid until losses exceed the volume given.
(2) If further fluid losses are unlikely to occur, give frusemide 20 mg IV.

Right heart failure

This occurs secondary to left heart failure, tricuspid regurgitation and chronic lung disease. Prevent hypoxia and hypercarbia.

Pulmonary embolism

See p. 112.

See p. 112.

Superior vena caval obstruction

During thoracic operations this may be due to a misplaced retractor, which should be repositioned.

Cardiac tamponade

When associated with hypotension, cardiac tamponade requires immediate drainage. Meanwhile, increase the inspired oxygen concentration and discontinue all myocardial-depressant drugs and volatile agents.

Decreased CVP

Check that the measuring device is correctly zeroed. If the CVP is low, the cause is hypovolaemia. Give fluids to raise the CVP.

Cardiac arrest

Diagnosis

(1) Absent carotid and femoral pulses; these may also be absent in severe hypotension. If the abdomen is open, impalpable aortic pulsation may be used to diagnose cardiac arrest.
(2) Asystole or ventricular fibrillation on the ECG. *NB*. Normal complexes may occur even though there is no cardiac output.

General treatment

(1) Inform the surgeon, and if necessary request his assistance.
(2) Note the time of the arrest and the state of the pupils.

(3) Strike the lower sternum with a closed fist. Sinus rhythm may be restored.
(4) Commence external cardiac massage. Depress the lower third of the sternum 4–5 cm 60 times per minute. Effective cardiac massage is best produced by keeping the arms fully extended and using the heels of the hands placed on top of one another. Cardiac massage may be stopped briefly to allow inflation of the chest, defibrillation and intracardiac injection of drugs. With these exceptions it should be used continuously until the patient is able to produce his own cardiac output or resuscitation is abandoned.
(5) Check the patency of the airway and inflate the lungs with 100% oxygen after every 5 cardiac compressions. It has recently been suggested that the lungs should be ventilated each time the heart is compressed.
(6) Check that the intravenous cannula is still functional. Give 8.4% sodium bicarbonate 100 ml stat. and then 5 ml per minute during resuscitation. Check the blood gases as soon as the opportunity arises, and if necessary modify the dose of sodium bicarbonate.
(7) Check the rhythm on an ECG.
(8) Disconnect unnecessary electrical apparatus and look for sources of electrocution.

Definitive treatment

Hypovolaemia

(1) Tell the surgeons to control major arterial or venous bleeding by clamping the appropriate vessels.
(2) Replace losses with an appropriate fluid.

Pneumothorax

See p. 110.

Air embolism

See p. 136.

Asystole

Try the following, allowing at least 1 minute after each injection for a beneficial effect.

(1) 10% calcium chloride 10 ml IV stat.; 5 ml increments may be given every 10 minutes.
(2) Adrenaline 1 mg IV; 0.5 mg increments may be given every 5 minutes.
(3) Intracardiac adrenaline 0.5–1 mg. Use a needle at least 4 cm long. Insert it in the fourth intercostal space at the mid-clavicular line and direct it backwards and cephalad at an angle of 45° to the sternum in the horizontal plane into the heart. Correct placement is indicated by the easy aspiration of blood.
(4) Isoprenaline 0.1–0.2 mg IV stat. This dose may be repeated after 5 minutes.
(5) Cardiac pacing. Use either an oesophageal pacing lead or a conventional temporary pacing lead placed in the right ventricle.

Coarse ventricular fibrillation (excluding digitalis-induced ventricular fibrillation)

This requires defibrillation.

(1) Cover the defibrillator pads with conducting jelly and charge the defibrillator with 100 J.
(2) Place one pad over ribs 2–4 in the right mid-clavicular line and the other over ribs 4–6 in the left mid-axillary line.
(3) Check that no-one (including yourself!) is touching the patient or the operating table.
(4) Discharge the shock.
(5) Allow 1 minute for spontaneous rhythm to return.
(6) If this fails, give 200, 300 and 400 J shocks at successive attempts.

Fine ventricular fibrillation

(1) Convert this to coarse ventricular fibrillation with adrenaline 0.5–1 mg IV or 10% calcium chloride 10 ml IV.
(2) Use the technique described above for coarse ventricular fibrillation.

Digitalis-induced ventricular fibrillation

(1) Use the technique described for coarse ventricular fibrillation, using low-energy shocks. Start with 10 J. Proceed to 20 and 40 J if necessary. If lower energies fail, 100 J may be required.
(2) Check the serum potassium and correct hyperkalaemia (see p. 18) or hypokalaemia (see p. 18).

Recurrent episodes of ventricular fibrillation

Correct the causes:

(1) Hypoxia: see pp. 110–113.
(2) Hypercarbia: see pp. 114–115.
(3) Metabolic acidosis: see p. 17.
(4) Electrolyte imbalance: see pp. 18–19.
(5) Predisposing rhythms (ventricular extrasystoles and ventricular tachycardia): see the section below.

Restoration of abnormal rhythm

(1) *Ventricular extrasystoles.* Lignocaine 1 mg/kg IV stat., followed by lignocaine infusion 4 mg per minute. If this fails try one of the following:
(a) practolol 5 mg IV slowly, plus increments up to 20 mg total dose;
(b) propranolol 1 mg IV slowly, plus increments up to 10 mg total dose;
(c) procainamide 100 mg IV slowly, plus increments up to 1 g total dose;
(d) mexiletine 150 mg IV;
(e) disopyramide 150 mg IV;
(f) phenytoin 100–200 mg.
   Beware of polypharmacy, as additive myocardial depression will occur.
(2) *Ventricular tachycardia.* Try any of the following:
(a) over-ride pacing if a pacing wire is *in situ*;
(b) defibrillation;
(c) practolol 5 mg IV, with increments up to 20 mg total dose;
(d) lignocaine 1 mg/kg IV stat., followed by an infusion at 4 mg per minute.

(3) *Supraventricular tachycardia*. Try the following:
    (a) carotid sinus or eyeball massage;
    (b) defibrillation;
    (c) practolol 5 mg IV, with increments up to 20 mg total dose.
(4) *Sinus bradycardia*. Try the following:
    (a) atropine 0.3–0.6 mg IV stat., with increments up to 1.8 mg;
    (b) cardiac pacing;
    (c) isoprenaline infusion (see Appendix 3).
(5) *Complete heart block*. Try the following:
    (a) cardiac pacing;
    (b) isoprenaline infusion (see Appendix 3).

Restoration of normal rhythm with hypotension

Try infusions of dopamine, dobutamine, isoprenaline or adrenaline (see Appendix 3).

Abandoning resuscitation

There are no rules. Make the decision having considered the following:

(1) Have you treated:
    (a) hypovolaemia?
    (b) hypoxia?
    (c) hypercarbia?
    (d) electrolyte imbalance?
    (e) metabolic acidosis?
    (f) pneumothorax?
    (g) air embolism?
(2) Have the depressant effects of anaesthetic drugs had time to wear off?
(3) Persistently fixed dilated pupils usually indicate that cerebral damage has occurred. This is not a reliable sign if atropine or trimetaphan has been given.

After-care

(1) Maintain the Pao_2 above 10 kPa, using IPPV if necessary.
(2) Check the serum electrolytes and acid–base status. Correct any abnormalities.
(3) Monitor the urine output. For causes and treatment of oliguria, see p. 138.

(4) Chest x-ray. Look for and treat fractured ribs or sternum, pneumothorax, haemothorax, haemopericardium or surgical emphysema. The chest x-ray may be delayed until the operation is completed provided the patient is closely monitored and you are aware that these complications may occur.
(5) Watch closely for signs of rarer complications, including gastric rupture, aortic rupture and lacerations of the spleen or liver.
(6) Give dexamethasone 10 mg IV stat. followed by 4 mg IV or IM 6-hourly in an attempt to control cerebral oedema. Avoid hypoxia and hypercarbia.

ECG changes

Ectopic rhythm

Atrial fibrillation

(1) Try increasing the inspired oxygen concentration.
(2) If the peripheral pulse rate is greater than 100 beats per minute give ouabain 0.25–0.5 mg IV slowly or digoxin 0.25 –0.5 mg IV slowly.

Atrial flutter

The treatment is the same as for atrial fibrillation (above).

Atrioventricular dissociation

(1) Treat possible causes, including hypocarbia and halothane relative overdose. Discontinue pancuronium or alcuronium.
(2) Give atropine 0.6 mg IV.

Nodal rhythm

(1) May be due to inadequate or excessive anaesthesia. Decide which is most likely and alter the depth of anaesthesia appropriately.
(2) Mild hypotension is common. If this is dangerous for the patient, give atropine 0.6 mg IV.

Ventricular extrasystoles

These require treatment only if they are multifocal, occur in runs or fall close to the T wave. Bigeminy also requires treatment.

(1) Treat possible causes, including hypoxia, hypercarbia, acidosis, halothane, hypertension, inadequate anaesthesia and digitalis toxicity (i.e. abnormal serum potassium).
(2) Give lignocaine 1 mg/kg IV. If ventricular extrasystoles recur, give a lignocaine infusion at a rate of 4 mg per minute (see Appendix 3).
(3) Propranolol 1 mg IV may also be used but is contraindicated in asthma and heart failure.

Supraventricular tachycardia

See p. 131.

Ventricular tachycardia

See p. 130.

Ventricular fibrillation

See p. 129.

Conduction defects

First-degree heart block

There is no specific treatment, but avoid hyperkalaemia, hypercarbia, hypoxia or increased vagal tone which may precipitate complete heart block.

Second-degree heart block

See 'First-degree heart block', above.

Complete heart block

Treat by cardiac pacing. Until this has been achieved, give an isoprenaline infusion (see Appendix 3).

Right bundle branch block

This rarely develops during anaesthesia but could indicate pulmonary embolism or myocardial ischaemia.

Left bundle branch block

This, too, is rare but could indicate myocardial ischaemia.

Change in level of ST segment

This always indicates myocardial ischaemia. Correct possible causes, including hypoxia (see pp. 110–113) and hypotension (see pp. 124–126).

Unequal ventilation of the lungs

Causes include the following.

Endobronchial intubation

See p. 110.

Collapse of a segment, lobe or whole lung

See p. 111.

Pneumothorax

See p. 110.

Difficulty inflating the chest

Ventilators with a pressure dial will show increased inflation pressure. Causes include the following.

Endobronchial intubation

See p. 110.

Obstruction or kinking of the endotracheal tube, catheter mount or anaesthetic circuit

See p. 110.

Bronchospasm

(1) Manually ventilate the patient with 100% oxygen. Use slow, gentle compressions of the bag to force air into the chest.
(2) Give aminophylline 4–6 mg/kg over 10 minutes or salbutamol 0.2 mg IV.
(3) If drug allergy is the cause, give chlorpheniramine 10 mg IV.

If these steps are unsuccessful, try:

(4) Adrenaline 0.25–0.5 mg IV slowly, or IM if the peripheral circulation is adequate.
(5) Ventilating with 10–15% ether in oxygen.
(6) Hydrocortisone 100 mg IV. This will not be effective for the first few hours.

Pneumothorax

See p. 110.

Increased end-tidal carbon dioxide tension

Increased end-tidal P_{CO_2} indicates hypoventilation. If the patient is breathing spontaneously, decrease the halothane or enflurane concentration. If this is not possible, change to IPPV. If the patient is being ventilated, increase the minute volume.

Decreased end-tidal carbon dioxide concentration

Causes include the following.

Hyperventilation

If the patient is being ventilated, decrease the minute volume.

Hypotension

See pp. 124–126.

Air embolism

Treat as follows:

(1) Prevent further air entering the circulation. Check drips. Press on the large veins which drain the operation site to raise the venous pressure. For other cases where venous compression is not possible, manually squeeze the reservoir bag against a closed valve. Ask the surgeon to cover the wound with wet swabs.
(2) Discontinue nitrous oxide. Ventilate with 100% oxygen.
(3) Place the patient in the left lateral head-down position.
(4) If hypotension occurs, give human plasma protein fraction.
(5) Attempt to aspirate the air through the CVP line if one is present.

See-saw respiration

See-saw respiration indicates respiratory obstruction; see p. 110.

Hiccoughs

Many remedies have been suggested but none is consistently effective:

(1) Pass a nasogastric tube and aspirate air.
(2) Increase the concentration of inhalational agents.
(3) Increase muscle relaxation but not at the expense of possible reversal problems.
(4) Stimulate the pharynx with a suction catheter.
(5) Manual hyperinflation of lungs for 20 seconds.
(6) Nikethamide 500 mg–1.25 g IV.
(7) Methylphenidate 20 mg IV.
(8) Check the serum electrolytes and acid–base status, and correct any abnormalities.
(9) Give the patient 6% carbon dioxide for 30 seconds.

Bubbling noises in the circuit

Mucus or blood in the endotracheal tube

Suck down the tube.

Water in the dependent loops of the circuit

Quickly disconnect the elephant tubing and drain the water. Remember to reconnect it afterwards.

Severe pulmonary oedema

(1) Check the fluid balance and reduce the rate of the infusion if overload has occurred.
(2) Give frusemide 40 mg IV.
(3) Ventilate the patient.
(4) Look for ECG abnormalities which can be treated (see pp. 132–134).

Increased core temperature

See p. 116.

Decreased core temperature

Reverse by:

(1) Increasing the theatre temperature.
(2) Warming intravenous fluids.
(3) Wrapping exposed areas of skin in cotton wool or blankets.

Increasing skin/core temperature difference

Causes include the following.

Peripheral cooling

Treatment is not necessary.

Inadequate anaesthesia

See p. 113.

Hypotension

See pp. 124–126.

Hypovolaemia

See p. 124.

Decreased urine output

Causes include the following.

Hypotension

See pp. 124–126.

Hypovolaemia

See p. 124.

Impending renal failure

(1) Correct hypotension and hypovolaemia.
(2) Stop enflurane and methoxyflurane because they are nephrotoxic.
(3) Frusemide 40 mg may promote an increased flow of dilute urine but should be given only as a last resort.

Raised intracranial pressure

Check that:

(1) The PaO_2 is normal or increased.
(2) The $PaCO_2$ is 3.5–4.0 kPa.
(3) The head is slightly raised.
(4) If the operation is not a craniotomy, that there are no localizing signs indicating haematoma formation. These may be masked by anaesthetic agents.
(5) Halothane is not being given to a spontaneously breathing patient.

Then give 20% mannitol 50 g over 20 minutes.

Failure to restart spontaneous respiration after suxamethonium

Causes include the following.

Hypocapnia

Failure to breathe may be caused by hypocapnia produced by excessive manual ventilation after intubating the patient. Give 5% carbon dioxide in oxygen.

Deficient or inactive plasma cholinesterase

Apnoea lasts several hours. Transfer the patient to an intensive care unit or recovery ward and ventilate until spontaneous respiration occurs. Avoid hyperventilation. If the patient has been given 100% oxygen, he will be awake. Explain to him that his breathing will return in a few hours. Use nitrous oxide and oxygen for ventilation; this will provide sedation without depressing respiration.

Dual block

Ventilate the patient as in the foregoing section until spontaneous respiration returns.

Failure to restart spontaneous respiration after non-depolarizing relaxants

Causes include the following.

Central nervous system depression

The patient has good muscle tone in his limbs but does not breathe. Causes include the following.

Overdose of analgesic

Give naloxone in 0.1 mg increments IV up to a total dose of 0.4 mg. If this is effective, the patient may have another episode of hypoventilation a few hours later when the naloxone wears off. Therefore, close postoperative monitoring is essential.

Overdose of halothane, enflurane or trichloroethylene

Allow adequate time for these agents to be excreted.

Hypocarbia

Measure the blood gases. If the Pa_{CO_2} is low, ventilate with 5% carbon dioxide in oxygen.

Inadequate hypoxic drive

This occurs in some chronic bronchitics. Ventilate with air.

Cerebrovascular accident

A cerebrovascular accident may occur during anaesthesia. Ventilate the patient until the diagnosis is confirmed.

Abnormal blood glucose

Measure the blood glucose, and if abnormal treat with either 25 ml 50% dextrose for hypoglycaemia or 12 units soluble insulin SC for hyperglycaemia.

Hangover from sedative premedicants

Try doxapram 1.0–1.5 mg/kg IV, followed by a doxapram infusion run at a rate of 3 mg per minute.

Hypothyroidism

Ventilate the patient and treat the hypothyroidism slowly.

Inadequate reversal of non-depolarizing relaxants

Causes include the following.

Inadequate dose of neostigmine

Give at least 5 mg IV accompanied by atropine 1.2 mg IV. There is no point giving any more neostigmine than 5 mg. Ventilate the patient until spontaneous respiration returns.

Potentiation of relaxant by electrolyte abnormalities

Check the serum sodium and potassium. If they are abnormal, correct slowly and ventilate the patient until spontaneous respiration returns.

Potentiation of relaxant by metabolic acidosis

Check the acid–base status, and if necessary give sodium bicarbonate (see p. 17).

Potentiation of relaxant by antibiotics

See Appendix 1 for relevant antibiotics. Sometimes calcium chloride 200–500 mg IV will reverse the block.

Potentiation of relaxant by trimetaphan or nitroglycerin

Ventilate the patient until spontaneous respiration returns.

Myasthenia gravis and myasthenic syndrome

These may be diagnosed only when the patient fails to breathe after reversal with neostigmine. Ventilate the patient until the diagnosis is made.

7

Problems occurring in the recovery period

Delayed awakening

Treat the cause.

Hypoxia

Hypoxia may be due to any of the following.

Inadequate ventilation

See pp. 144–147.

Pneumothorax

See p. 110.

Atelectasis

Treat with physiotherapy and give 40% oxygen via a face mask.

Collapse of a lobe or a whole lung

Bronchoscopy is indicated.

Hypotension

See p. 153.

Myocardial failure

See p. 112.

Pulmonary embolism

See p. 112.

Malignant hyperpyrexia

See p. 112.

Acid aspiration

See p. 108.

Hypercarbia

Hypercarbia may be due to either of the following.

Inadequate ventilation

See pp. 144–147.

Malignant hyperpyrexia

See p. 112.

Continued action of sedative premedication

Try giving doxapram 1.0–1.5 mg/kg IV. If this is successful, use a doxapram infusion at a rate of 3 mg per minute until the premedication has worn off. In elderly patients, hyoscine (sometimes) and atropine (rarely) cause delayed recovery. Their effects may be reversed with physostigmine 2 mg IV.

Relative overdose of halothane, enflurane or trichloroethylene

Be patient and these gases will be exhaled.

Relative overdose of narcotic analgesic

Give naloxone 0.1–0.4 mg IV. Watch the patient carefully because naloxone is short-acting and another dose may be required after a few hours.

Hypoglycaemia

If the blood sugar is low, give 50% dextrose 25 ml into a large vein.

Hyperglycaemia

If the blood sugar is greater than 20 mmol/l, give soluble insulin 12 units SC. Check the blood sugar again after 1 hour; if it is still raised, an insulin infusion should be started.

Cerebrovascular accident

Give dexamethasone 10 mg IV.

Fat embolism

This may occur in trauma patients, particularly those who have had a long bone fracture. Check the blood gases and ensure adequate oxygenation.

Inadequate ventilation

Inadequate reversal of muscle relaxants

See pp. 140–141.

Obstructed upper respiratory tract

(1) The patient should be lying in the semi-prone position.
(2) Clear the pharynx of blood and secretions. Check for foreign bodies.
(3) Push the vertical ramus of the mandible forwards and slightly upwards.
(4) Insert an oropharyngeal or nasopharyngeal airway if the patient will tolerate it.

Larynospasm

(1) Examine the vocal cords and remove blood, vomit and secretions.
(2) Support the jaw and give the patient 100% oxygen via a face mask.

(3) If the spasm does not resolve and the patient is becoming cyanosed, give thiopentone and suxamethonium, and reintubate. Prior to extubation give 100% oxygen for at least 3 minutes. Watch the patient carefully, as laryngospasm may recur.

Facial and/or laryngeal swelling

Secure the airway by reintubating the patient if severe obstruction is imminent. Specific treatment should then be given. If the swelling is minimal, specific treatments may be tried prior to intubation, as follows.

Traumatic intubation

Give dexamethasone 10 mg IV and humidified oxygen via a face mask.

Acute fluid changes associated with extubation

These patients often have low plasma proteins. The swelling will gradually resolve without treatment. Try raising serum proteins with human plasma protein fraction or albumin.

Allergic reaction

Decide which drug or fluid has precipitated the reaction and discontinue it. Give chlorpheniramine 10 mg IV. Severe reactions may require adrenaline 0.25–0.5 mg IM.

Pregnancy

Laryngeal swelling occurs in pregnancy and is often associated with pre-eclampsia. Usually it resolves fairly quickly after delivery.

Sporadic or hereditary angioneurotic oedema

Various treatments have been suggested. The most useful are fresh-frozen plasma 6 packs IV, adrenaline 0.5 mg SC or chlorpheniramine 10 mg IV.

Air

Surgical emphysema may be palpable in the neck. Give 40% oxygen. If the emphysema is severe and involves the chest wall, insertion of chest drains connected to an underwater seal may be of long-term benefit.

Surgical trauma

Give dexamethasone 10 mg IV and humidified oxygen via a face mask.

Bronchospasm

See p. 135.

Lack of stimulation

Some patients forget to breathe unless they are verbally encouraged to do so.

Central nervous system depression

See pp. 139–140.

Splinting of the diaphragm or thoracic cage

Treat the cause.

Pain

Pain is best treated with an intravenous drug; e.g. dilute 10 mg morphine up to 10 ml in physiological saline solution giving a concentration of 1 mg/ml. Give 1 mg increments, watching for respiratory depression until the pain is relieved.

Gastric distension

Aspirate air and fluid from the stomach via a nasogastric tube. Leave the nasogastric tube on free drainage.

Tight circumferential dressings

These should be loosened.

Surgical emphysema

See 'Air', above.

Cyanosis

Central cyanosis

Central cyanosis is due to hypoxia (or methaemoglobinaemia).

Hypoxia

See pp. 142–143.

Diffusion hypoxia

Give 40% oxygen via a face mask.

Methaemoglobinaemia

Give 1% methylene blue 1 mg/kg IV.

Peripheral cyanosis

Causes include the following.

Hypoxia

See pp. 142–143.

Cold

Warm the patient slowly by covering him with warm blankets. Use a space blanket to prevent further cooling. Warm infusion fluids. Give 40% oxygen via a face mask.

Pre-existing poor peripheral circulation

Treatment is unnecessary.

Hypotension

See p. 153.

Hypovolaemia

See p. 153.

Stridor

Treat the cause.

Laryngeal obstruction

Examine the larynx and remove blood clot, secretions, vomitus or a foreign body.

Laryngeal swelling

See pp. 145–146.

Hyperventilation

Treat the cause.

Anxiety

Reassure the patient. If this fails, give diazepam 2–5 mg IV.

Pain

See p. 146.

Hypercarbia

Inadequate ventilation

See pp. 144–147.

Malignant hyperpyrexia

See pp. 112–113.

Metabolic acidosis

Diabetic ketoacidosis

Treatment includes insulin, fluid and potassium. You will probably require the assistance of a physician when managing this
problem. See also Chapter 9.

Other causes

Give sodium bicarbonate (see p. 17).

Central nervous system damage

Ventilate the patient until the diagnosis is confirmed.

Abnormal muscle movements

Inadequate reversal of muscle relaxant

See pp. 139 and 140–141.

Shivering

Due to peroperative cooling

See p. 147.

Halothane 'shakes'

Give 40% oxygen via a face mask. Severe trismus may prevent
maintenance of a patent airway. Try inserting a nasopharyngeal
airway. If this fails, give thiopentone and suxamethonium, and
reintubate the patient. If the spasm lasts longer than 5 minutes,
give methylphenidate 20 mg IV. Occasionally persistent sinus
tachycardia, nodal tachycardia or ventricular extrasystoles occur
with the halothane 'shakes'. Treat with oxprenolol 1 mg IV.

Epidural 'shakes'

These sometimes occur after a top-up of bupivacaine. Reassure
the patient. No treatment is required.

Convulsions

Treat the following abnormalities, which may occur alone or in combination.

Hypoxia

Give 100% oxygen via a face mask. If necessary, give thiopentone and suxamethonium, and reintubate the patient.

Hypocarbia

Give 5% carbon dioxide in oxygen for 5 minutes.

Pyrexia

Cool the patient with a fan and tepid sponging.

Hypoglycaemia

Give 50% dextrose 25 ml into a large vein.

Hypocalcaemia

Give 10% calcium chloride 10 ml IV.

Withdrawal of anticonvulsants preoperatively

Give diazepam 10 mg IV. If this fails, give thiopentone and suxamethonium, and reintubate. Control further fits with tubocurarine and thiopentone. Start the patient's normal treatment regimen as soon as possible, using the intramuscular route if necessary.

CNS disease (e.g. oedema, embolism, tumour, haematoma)

Give thiopentone and suxamethonium, intubate the patient and hyperventilate with 40% oxygen. Give dexamethasone 10 mg IV. A haematoma should be treated surgically.

Water intoxication

Give frusemide 20 mg IV.

Eclampsia

This can occur immediately following delivery. Give a diazepam infusion at 20 mg per hour and hydrallazine 20 mg IV followed by an infusion (see Appendix 3). Maintain the urine output with intermittent doses of frusemide 20 mg IV. Do clotting studies, as disseminated intravascular coagulation may occur.

Malignant hypertension

Give diazoxide 300 mg IV and diazepam 10 mg IV.

Restlessness

Restlessness may be due to any of the following.

Pain

Give an intravenous analgesic (see p. 146).

Hypoxia

Give 40% oxygen via a face mask (see pp. 147–148).

Respiratory obstruction

Clear pharyngeal secretions and support the jaw. Reintubate if necessary.

Hypotension

Treat the cause (see p. 153).

Anxiety

Reassure the patient. If necessary, give diazepam 2–5 mg IV.

Ketamine hallucinations

Allow the patient to recover in a quiet room without being disturbed by nurses or medical staff.

Hypertension

Treat the cause.

Pain

See p. 146. Remember that pain may also be caused by a full bladder.

Hypoxia

See pp. 142–143.

Hypercarbia

Reintubate and gently hyperventilate the patient. Rapid reduction in $PaCO_2$ may cause hypotension.

Fluid overload

Slow down the intravenous infusion.

Cerebral oedema

Reintubate and hyperventilate the patient so that the $PaCO_2$ is 3.5–4.0 kPa. Ensure that the PaO_2 is 14–16 kPa. Give mannitol 1 g/kg IV over 20 minutes.

Vasopressor infusion

This may inadvertently have been left switched on.

Aortic embolism or thrombosis

This very rare problem causes absent femoral pulses. The treatment is surgical.

Undiagnosed phaeochromocytoma

See Chapter 9.

Hypotension

Causes include the following.

Hypovolaemia

Check the fluid balance and replace fluids appropriately. Beware of occult bleeding due to a slipped ligature.

Pain

See p. 146. Atropine 0.3 mg IV may also be required.

Drug-induced

Check that halothane or enflurane and hypotensive infusions are switched off. Administration of narcotic analgesics sometimes causes hypotension. Up to 500 ml physiological saline solution may be required to raise the BP.

Adrenal insufficiency

Give hydrocortisone 100 mg IV.

Myocardial failure

Give frusemide 40 mg IV and consider giving ouabain 0.25–0.5 mg IV slowly for rapid digitalization.

Dysrhythmias

See pp. 132–134.

Cardiac arrest

See pp. 127–132.

Dysrhythmias and conduction defects

See pp. 132–134.

Nausea and vomiting

Treat the cause.

Respiratory obstruction

See pp. 144–146.

Pharyngeal irritation

This may be due to blood, secretions, vomit or other foreign bodies. These should be removed.

Anaesthetic agents or narcotic analgesics

Give prochlorperazine 12.5 mg IM. Prevent excessive movement by calming words or specific treatment (see pp. 149–151). Movement aggravates the nausea and vomiting caused by morphine. NB. Pain itself can cause vomiting.

Gastric distension

Aspirate air and fluid from the stomach via a nasogastric tube. Leave the nasogastric tube on free drainage.

Intraperitoneal operations

Give prochlorperazine 12.5 mg IM.

Cerebral oedema

Ensure that the PaO_2 is 14–16 kPa and the $PaCO_2$ is 3.5–4.0 kPa. Give mannitol 1 g/kg over 20 minutes. If necessary, reintubate and hyperventilate the patient.

Pain

Treat with one of the following methods.

Local anaesthesia

If an epidural has been used for the operation, continue to top it up for postoperative pain relief.

Entonox

This mixture of 50% nitrous oxide in oxygen may be used for short-term reversible pain relief equivalent to morphine 10 mg IM when other analgesics are contraindicated (e.g. postoperative respiratory depression, head injuries).

Intravenous analgesia

This provides rapid pain relief. See p. 146 for technique.

Intramuscular analgesia

This should be prescribed for use in the ward.

Sweating

Hypoxia

See pp. 142–143.

Hypercarbia

See pp. 144–147.

Pain

See the foregoing main section.

Vasovagal reaction

Give atropine 0.6 mg IV.

Malignant hyperpyrexia

See pp. 112–113.

Increased core temperature

See p. 116.

Hypoglycaemia

Give 50% dextrose 25 ml IV.

Excessive bleeding from the wound

Inadequate surgical haemostasis

This may be due to failure to tie a bleeding vessel or a slipped ligature.

Transfusion reaction

See p. 117.

Platelet deficiency

See p. 119.

Clotting factor deficiency

See p. 119.

Ionized calcium deficiency

See p. 119.

Increased capillary fragility

See p. 119.

Disseminated intravascular coagulation

See p. 119.

Fibrinolysis

See p. 120.

8

Anaesthesia for specific procedures

Some anaesthetic techniques for emergency surgical procedures are described below, in alphabetical order. The general advice given in Chapter 5 should always be followed and used in conjunction with the suggestions made in this chapter. Several techniques may be available and equally acceptable for each operation. Use the technique with which you are most familiar, and ask for help if you feel unable to give a safe anaesthetic on your own.

Angiography (except carotid angiography)

Use a technique similar to that described for carotid angiography (see p. 159). Fentanyl may be used to provide analgesia.

Bronchoscopy, fibreoptic

Local anaesthesia (see pp. 59–60) is often sufficient. For general anaesthesia, induce with Althesin, etomidate or methohexitone. Paralyse with suxamethonium and intubate with the largest endotracheal tube which can be passed. Give atropine. Maintain anaesthesia with increments of the induction agent, and maintain paralysis with intermittent suxamethonium or a suxamethonium infusion (see Appendix 3). Ventilate the patient with 100% oxygen via the endotracheal tube. The bronchoscope may be passed through the rubber bung in the connector, which should already have had a suitably sized hole cut in it.

Bronchoscopy, rigid

Use local anaesthesia (see pp. 59–60) for frail patients and those in whom general anaesthesia is contraindicated. Insufflate oxygen to maintain good oxygenation.

For general anaesthesia induce with Althesin, etomidate or methohexitone. Paralyse with suxamethonium and give atropine. Maintain anaesthesia with increments of the induction agent, and paralysis with intermittent suxamethonium or a suxamethonium infusion (see Appendix 3). Use an injection device to ventilate the patient with 100% oxygen.

Rarely, some foreign bodies act as a ball-valve. It is dangerous to paralyse and ventilate in these circumstances. Induce deep anaesthesia, via a face mask, with oxygen, nitrous oxide and halothane. Maintain anaesthesia by allowing the patient to breathe oxygen and halothane insufflated down the bronchoscope.

Caesarian section

Having ensured that the stomach is as empty as possible, premedicate with magnesium trisilicate mixture 20 ml on the ward followed by 20 ml immediately before induction. Use a wedge to achieve a lateral tilt of 15°. Preoxygenate the patient and induce anaesthesia with hyoscine 0.6 mg IV, thiopentone 250–300 mg IV and suxamethonium 100 mg IV as consciousness is lost. Apply cricoid pressure. Intubate the patient.

Maintain relaxation with a suxamethonium infusion (see Appendix 3), and anaesthesia with oxygen and nitrous oxide in a ratio of 2:1, supplemented by 0.2% trichloroethylene. The high concentration of oxygen provides optimal oxygenation of the fetus prior to delivery. There is a 5% risk of maternal awareness, but this is not always unpleasant and is outweighed by benefits to the baby. The ratio of oxygen to nitrous oxide may be reversed after delivery of the baby.

When the baby has been delivered, give syntocinon 5 i.u. IV followed by a syntocinon infusion (10 i.u. in 500 ml dextrose) for several hours postoperatively.

Some obstetricians are unhappy unless ergometrine 250 µg IV is given. Ergometrine causes vomiting and should be avoided if possible. It is definitely contraindicated if there is a history of hypertension, pre-eclampsia or eclampsia.

If an epidural has already been given for pain relief during labour, it may be possible to top it up so that the level reaches T6 and perform the caesarian section under epidural. The surgeon must be reminded to be gentle with the bowels and to suck the liquor away quickly so that it does not reach the diaphragm. If these precautions are not observed, the patient may become nauseated and vomit. Syntocinon should be used as the oxytocic.

Even if there is no time to top up the epidural, it can still be used to provide postoperative pain relief.

Cardioversion

Check the serum potassium and correct it if it is abnormal. Note whether the patient is taking digitalis. If so, smaller shocks should be used by the doctor performing the cardioversion. Check that resuscitation equipment is available. Preoxygenate for 3 minutes.

Induce anaesthesia with the standard induction dose of Althesin, etomidate or methohexitone. Insert an airway. Cardiovert the patient. Then give 100% oxygen until the patient awakes. Rarely, if multiple shocks are given, an incremental dose of the induction agent may be required. Some anaesthetists rely on the amnesic effect of 5–10 mg diazepam for cardioversion.

Carotid angiography

The technique is the same as that described for CAT scanning (see p. 160). It is important to hyperventilate the patient in order that the cerebral blood vessels are constricted, as this facilitates the interpretation of the films. After the patient has been hyperventilated, a low concentration of halothane or trichloroethylene may be used to deepen the anaesthesia. This is sometimes necessary because the contrast medium causes pain when it is injected.

Carotid endarterectomy

Many techniques have been suggested but none is outstandingly better than the rest. Some surgeons prefer to work under local anaesthesia. The anaesthetic technique should provide good oxygenation, normocarbia and a normal BP or mild hypertension. Induce anaesthesia with thiopentone. Give atropine 0.6 mg IV to protect against bradycardia and hypotension when the carotid sinus is manipulated. Spontaneous respiration with halothane or IPPV with alcuronium, fentanyl and low concentrations of halothane are both successful techniques. Monitor the arterial blood gases and BP. Some surgeons measure the stump pressure or record the electroencephalogram to assess the adequacy of the cerebral circulation.

Postoperatively give 40% oxygen via a face mask. Monitor the BP and ECG. Hypertension should be treated with a trimetaphan infusion (see Appendix 3). Hypotension should be treated with a phenylephrine infusion (see Appendix 3). Dysrhythmias may also require treatment (see pp. 132–134).

CAT scanning

Anaesthesia may be required to keep unco-operative patients still. Sedation is contraindicated because it may depress respiration. As there is often raised intracranial pressure, it is best to hyperventilate the patient with nitrous oxide and oxygen so that the $PaCO_2$ is 3.5–4.0 kPa. Prevent coughing, straining and vomiting at induction. Use a non-kinking tube. Position the connector so that the elephant tubing will not get tangled with the scanner. Check that the tubing is long enough to allow for movements of the table. Scanning rooms are often cold; cover the patient with blankets unless this interferes with the procedure. Decide whether you will wear a lead apron and stay with the patient or whether you will interrupt the procedure at frequent intervals to allow you to check his BP. If you decide on the latter course, it is essential to monitor the ECG so that you can watch the trace from outside the scanning room. It is also important that you are able to see the patient's chest moving.

Craniotomy

Whatever the reason for the operation, it is important not to raise the intracranial pressure. Use a technique similar to that described for CAT scanning (see the foregoing section). Reflex hypertension may occur as a protective mechanism if the intracranial pressure is raised secondary to a subdural or extradural haematoma. Maintain this BP until the clot has been evacuated.

For other craniotomies, a hypotensive technique is useful. Reduce the BP with a trimetaphan infusion or sodium nitroprusside infusion (see Appendix 3). Trimetaphan, but not sodium nitroprusside, may be used before the cranium is opened. Mannitol also may be given to reduce the intracranial pressure. Halothane 0.5% may be given to patients with raised intracranial pressure after the $PaCO_2$ has been lowered to 3.5–4.0 kPa. Analgesic agents are best avoided because they may confuse signs of raised intracranial pressure postoperatively. Remember that trimetaphan causes fixed dilated pupils for several hours postoperatively.

Electroconvulsive therapy

This is not a true emergency. The patient should be adequately starved. Preoxygenate the patient. Give thiopentone 150–250 mg IV, suxamethonium 25–45 mg IV and atropine 1.0 mg IV. Insert a rubber mouth gag (or an airway if the patient is edentulous). When the fasciculations have stopped, the shock may be given. Ventilate the patient via a face mask with 100% oxygen until spontaneous respiration returns. The doses of thiopentone and suxamethonium will depend on the size and fitness of the patient. Note how well the convulsion is modified; this will help the next anaesthetist who is asked to anaesthetize the patient.

Evacuation of retained products of conception

Remember that there is an increased risk of regurgitation even in the early stages of pregnancy. The same technique may be used as that described for caesarian section.

Eye surgery

Closed eye surgery

Suitable conditions are provided by allowing the patient to breathe halothane spontaneously. Atropine 0.6 mg IV should be given to protect against the oculocardiac reflex.

Open eye surgery

The eye may be opened at operation or be open due to a penetrating eye injury. It is important not to raise the intraocular pressure. Premedication should include an antiemetic (e.g. cyclizine 50 mg IM). If there is a penetrating eye injury, induce anaesthesia with thiopentone, atropine and pancuronium (see p. 83). If the eye is closed at induction, use the standard technique (see pp. 81–83). Whichever method is used, it is important to prevent straining, coughing and vomiting.

Ventilate the patient during the procedure. The agents used do not matter provided that the BP remains normal or slightly reduced, there is good oxygenation and the patient is slightly hypocarbic. Monitor the BP and ECG. The atropine should protect against the oculocardiac reflex, but if it does occur give more atropine up to a total dose of 1.2 mg.

The patient should be well sedated but able to protect his own airway at the end of the operation. Coughing should, if possible, be avoided at extubation. This implies that the patient should be extubated as soon as possible after spontaneous respiration has returned, even if the cough reflex is not present. Turn the patient on his side and suck out the pharynx prior to reversal and extubation.

Laparoscopy

Use a suxamethonium drip supplemented with fentanyl and hyperventilate the patient. Increased inflation pressures will be required when the abdomen is distended with gas. Check the blood pressure frequently. Hypotension may be due to abdominal overdistension or, rarely, a gas embolism. The intraperitoneal pressure should never exceed 30 mmHg. A torch or other means of illumination should be used to check the patient's colour, etc., when the theatre is darkened during laparoscopy.

Laparotomy

Some degree of muscle relaxation is always required. If a Pfannensteil incision is used, a suxamethonium infusion will provide adequate relaxation. For other incisions it is usually necessary to use a non-depolarizing relaxant.

Maxillofacial surgery

Use a non-kinking tube. Position the connector so that the elephant tubing is placed away from the operating field. Remember that maintaining the airway and intubation may be difficult. Choose your technique accordingly. Use a throat pack to protect the upper airway. Do not forget to remove it.

Oesophagoscopy

Provide continuous relaxation with intermittent suxamethonium or a suxamethonium infusion (see Appendix 3) and anaesthesia via an endotracheal tube with oxygen and nitrous oxide. Supplement nitrous oxide anaesthesia with fentanyl or an inhalational agent.

Renal transplantation

Note the problems caused by renal failure (see Chapter 9). Use IPPV. Small doses of pancuronium should be used to provide muscle relaxation. Maintain anaesthesia with fentanyl or low concentrations of halothane. Avoid hypotension. When the vascular anastomoses have been completed, give frusemide 250 mg IV to induce a diuresis. Give fluids cautiously, replacing only losses due to starvation, insensible loss and haemorrhage.

Reverse anaesthesia with normal doses of neostigmine and atropine. Postoperatively give 40% oxygen via a face mask.

Thoracotomy

Employ a double-lumen tube (see p. 72). Always ventilate the patient when the pleura is open. Provide muscle relaxation with a non-depolarizing relaxant and supplement nitrous oxide anaesthesia with an analgesic or inhalational agent. When one lung is collapsed, monitor the blood gases to ensure that ventilation is adequate. To reduce the inflation pressure, decrease the tidal volume and increase the rate of ventilation. Minimize hypoxia by insufflating oxygen at a rate of 3 litres per minute into the collapsed lung. Prior to closure of the chest manually hyperinflate the lungs several times to reinflate them. This is particularly important if a chest drain has not been inserted.

9

Anaesthesia in relation to specific conditions

In this chapter are discussed briefly, in alphabetical order, conditions and symptoms which have particular implications for anaesthesia. Many of these entries include associated factors, discussed under other headings; these are printed in italics, giving either the full term (e.g. 'Addison's disease') or the index word (e.g. 'megaloblastic anaemia').

Achalasia. The risk of regurgitation is increased. Malnutrition may cause protein deficiency and altered drug binding. Preoperatively, pass a nasogastric or stomach tube into the oesophagus and aspirate its contents.

Achondroplasia. Inability to extend the cervical spine together with abnormal bony development of the skull may make intubation difficult. Thoracic abnormalities may restrict respiration (see *Restrictive lung disease*).

Acidosis, renal tubular, causes hypokalaemia, nephrocalcinosis and hence *renal impairment* or *failure* and *osteomalacia.*

Acrocephalosyndactyly. Intubation may be difficult. These patients sometimes have congenital heart disease and raised *intracranial pressure.*

Acrocyanosis. This disease is innocuous. It may obscure peripheral cyanosis of a more serious nature.

Acromegaly. Intubation is often difficult. The collateral circulation from the ulnar artery may be inadequate for safe cannulation of the radial artery. Kyphosis (see *Kyphoscoliosis*), *hypertension, cardiomyopathy, congestive cardiac failure, cerebrovascular accidents* and *diabetes mellitus* are associated with acromegaly. Late in the disease adrenal insufficiency (see *Addison's disease*) and *hypothyroidism* may occur. Acromegalics may be extremely sensitive to opiates.

Actinomycosis. If it occurs in the face, intubation may be difficult. Oral infections may spread to the lungs and cause severe *pneumonia*.

Adams–Stokes attacks may be due to brief episodes of ventricular asystole, tachycardia or fibrillation. Transient complete heart block is also a cause. A diagnosis should be made, if possible, by continuous ECG monitoring. If there is insufficient time to pace the patient preoperatively, prepare resuscitation drugs, a defibrillator and equipment for temporary pacing in theatre.

Addiction, alcohol. Associated diseases include *diabetes mellitus*, *cirrhosis*, chronic *pancreatitis*, malnutrition, pulmonary infection secondary to aspiration, *cardiomyopathy*, megaloblastic *anaemia* and peripheral *neuropathy*. Fluid balance and electrolytes may be abnormal. The patient may be overhydrated or dehydrated. Maintain good oxygenation because alcoholics have a decreased cerebral tolerance to hypoxia. The problem is aggravated because mild hypoxia is common due to shunting in the liver. Premedicate with intravenous Parenterovite I and II and a normal dose of diazepam. Induction may be stormy, and increased doses of thiopentone or halothane should be used. The response to suxamethonium may be prolonged. If a non-depolarizing relaxant is used, choose pancuronium. Be prepared for difficulty with reversal if the electrolytes have not been adequately corrected. Use fentanyl or halothane to supplement nitrous oxide anaesthesia. Use decreased doses of morphine for postoperative pain. Watch for signs of withdrawal, which should be treated with an infusion of 0.8% chlormethiazole.

The above remarks apply to chronic alcoholism without recent intake of alcohol. If the patient is intoxicated, stomach emptying will be delayed. Reduced doses of induction and maintenance agents will be required. Peripheral vasodilatation will reduce the patient's tolerance to cold, myocardial-depressant drugs and haemorrhage. Recovery may be prolonged. Watch for hypoglycaemia during and after the operation.

Use local anaesthetics with caution because liver disease may cause clotting abnormalities. Intoxicated patients tend to be unco-operative.

Addiction, amphetamines. Chronic intake causes a decreased requirement for thiopentone. There is a poor response to vasopressors. Hypotension should be treated with a noradrenaline infusion (see Appendix 3). Dependence is psychological. Chlorpromazine may be required during withdrawal. Acute intake preoperatively may cause an increased requirement for thiopentone, hypertension, pyrexia, convulsions and dysrhythmias. Halothane is contraindicated because it may aggravate dysrhythmias.

Addiction, barbiturates. The patient should be sedated preoperatively. Increased doses of thiopentone or methohexitone are required for induction. An inhalational induction requires normal doses. Barbiturates should be withdrawn slowly. Acute withdrawal may be fatal.

Addiction, cannabis. Dependence is psychological. Cannabis consumption is often associated with chronic *bronchitis* and possibly liver disease. Anaesthesia is usually uneventful although a decreased dose of thiopentone is often sufficient. Acute intake causes a sinus tachycardia.

Addiction, cocaine. Premedicate the patient with diazepam. Avoid halothane, which may cause dysrhythmias or hypotension. Hypotension is resistant to treatment with vasopressors.

Addiction, glue. May cause aplastic *anaemia, hepatic failure* and *renal failure.* Anaemia and clotting abnormalities may require preoperative correction.

Addiction, glutethimide. The problems are the same as for barbiturate *addiction.*

Addiction, heroin. See *Addiction, morphine.*

Addiction, isopropyl alcohol. *Hepatic* and *renal impairment* may occur. A metabolic acidosis is common.

Addiction, LSD. Narcotic analgesics and suxamethonium may be potentiated. LSD is a mild *MAOI. Hepatic* and *renal impairment* may occur. Withdrawal symptoms and 'flash-backs' due to the stress of surgery should be treated with chlorpromazine or barbiturates.

Addiction, meprobamate. An increased dose of thiopentone may be required for induction. The circulatory reflexes are depressed, rendering the patient particularly susceptible to hypotension with IPPV, the head-up position or hypovolaemia.

Addiction, mescaline. Premedicate the patient with diazepam. There are no anaesthetic problems. Dependence is psychological.

Addiction, methyl alcohol. The problems are the same as for isopropyl alcohol *addiction.*

Addiction, methyprylone. The problems as the same as for barbiturate *addiction.*

Addiction, morphine. Associated diseases include infective *endocarditis, pneumonia,* atelectasis, septic pulmonary infarcts, *hepatic impairment, hepatitis* B and *syphilis.* Give the normal maintenance dose as premedication. Hypotension peroperatively may be due to inadequate analgesia or relative adrenal insufficiency. The latter should be treated with hydrocortisone. Prophylactic steroids are not necessary. Postoperatively give the normal maintenance dose of morphine or methadone 10 mg IM. If the methadone analgesia is insufficient, give 5–10 mg IM 1 hour after the initial dose. Repeat the total dose of methadone 12-hourly. Morphine addicts may plead pain as an excuse for another dose of morphine.

Recently withdrawn patients should be given only methadone 10–20 mg IM as premedication and for postoperative pain. Completely withdrawn patients should never be given morphine. Give pentazocine 30–60 mg IM 4-hourly for pain relief. Local anaesthesia may be suitable for anaesthesia and postoperative pain relief.

Addiction, psilocybin. The problems are the same as for LSD *addiction,* but suxamethonium is not potentiated.

Addison's disease may be associated with pernicious *anaemia,* thyroiditis or *hypothyroidism.* Causes include primary adrenal failure and *hypopituitarism.* Check for hypoglycaemia, hyponatraemia and hyperkalaemia. Correct if necessary. *Steroid* cover should be given. These patients tend to be relatively hypotensive and are prone to postural hypotension and hypovolaemia. They are sensitive to barbiturates, narcotic analgesics and sedatives, which should be used in reduced doses.

Adrenal insufficiency. See *Addison's disease.*

Adrenogenital syndrome. All cases require *steroid* cover. Some are salt losing. Give fludrocortisone 0.05–0.1 mg orally to cover the operation and an anti-emetic (e.g. cyclizine 50 mg IM) to prevent further sodium loss. Give physiological saline solution peroperatively.

Agammaglobulinaemia. The patient may require *steroid* cover. Use aseptic techniques to prevent infection.

Agranulocytosis. These patients should be adequately hydrated and maintained at a normal temperature. Avoid chlorpromazine and sulphonamides, which may cause the disease.

Albers–Schönberg disease. These patients are anaemic and pathological fractures are common. Move the unconscious patient gently.

Albinism may, rarely, be associated with *hypopituitarism*.

Albright–Butler syndrome is associated with *renal impairment*.

Albright's osteodystrophy. Hypocalcaemia may cause convulsions or inadequate reversal of neuromuscular-blocking agents.

Alcoholism. See *Addiction, alcohol*.

Aldosteronism, primary. The untreated disease is associated with electrolyte abnormalities, particularly hypokalaemia. Potassium chloride 2–6 g daily for several days preoperatively may be required to correct the deficit. Spironolactone treatment may cause hyponatraemia. Associated diseases include *hypertension, renal impairment, congestive cardiac failure* and *cerebrovascular accidents*. When the tumour is handled, there may be severe hypertension and temporary cortical insufficiency. Treat with a trimetaphan infusion (Appendix 3) and hydrocortisone.

Aldosteronism, secondary, is usually secondary to renal damage. It may be associated with *congestive cardiac failure* and *hepatic failure*.

Alport syndrome. The most significant problem is *renal failure*.

Alström syndrome consists of *obesity, renal failure* and *diabetes mellitus*.

Alveolitis, allergic, causes *restrictive lung disease*. Steroid therapy is often given to severe cases, who may require high concentrations of oxygen during anaesthesia.

Alveolitis, fibrosing, often causes *congestive cardiac failure*. *Steroids* are used for treatment. Ensure adequate oxygenation throughout anaesthesia.

Amoebiasis causes anaemia, electrolyte deficiencies and *intestinal obstruction*. Maintain good oxygenation, as the lungs may be involved.

Amyloidosis. Associated diseases include *hypertension, congestive cardiac failure*, conduction defects and dysrhythmias, *renal failure* and *hepatic failure*. *Steroids* are used for its treatment. Delayed gastric emptying is common. Macroglossia may hinder intubation. Avoid skin shearing, which may cause bullae.

Amyotonia congenita. These patients are extremely sensitive to respiratory-depressant drugs. Use thiopentone and narcotic analgesics in reduced doses. Muscle relaxants should be avoided if possible.

Amyotrophic lateral sclerosis. See *Motor neuron disease*.

Anaemia, aplastic. Fresh blood or platelet transfusions may be necessary preoperatively. Use aseptic techniques to avoid infection. *Steroid* cover may be required.

Anaemia, autoimmune haemolytic. The warm antibody type is associated with *steroid therapy* and prolonged apnoea after suxamethonium. The cold antibody type requires that the patient be kept at a normal temperature and washed red cells be used for transfusion. Monitor the temperature because hyperthermia may occur. The drug-induced type is associated with *steroid therapy*. Avoid precipitating drugs.

Anaemia, megaloblastic, should be corrected with whole blood preoperatively only if absolutely necessary. If congestive cardiac failure is present, an exchange transfusion should be performed. The toxicity of sodium nitroprusside is increased. Associated diseases include alcohol *addiction*, *Crohn's disease* and *blind loop syndrome*.

Anaemia, microangiopathic, is usually treated with heparin and *steroids*.

Anaemia, pernicious, may be associated with *thyroiditis*, *hypothyroidism*, *Addison's disease* and *hypoparathyroidism*.

Anaemia, sideroblastic, may be associated with respiratory insufficiency and *hepatic impairment*.

Anaemia, target cell. See *Thalassaemia*.

Analbuminaemia. These patients are very sensitive to thiopentone and tubocurarine, which should be avoided or used in greatly reduced doses.

Analphalipoproteinaemia. These patients are anaemic and thrombocytopenic. They are prone to premature *ischaemic heart disease*. Use muscle relaxants with care because the patient may respond abnormally.

Andersen's disease is associated with *hepatic failure* and hypoglycaemia.

Aneurysm, leaking aortic. This is a disease of old age and therefore may be associated with *hypertension*, *ischaemic heart disease*, chronic *bronchitis* and *emphysema*. Under local anaesthesia, insert two large peripheral cannulae, a radial artery cannula and central venous line. Give cross-matched fresh whole blood to avoid clotting problems due to massive blood transfusion. Use a warming blanket. Transfuse the patient to a normal systolic BP. Induce anaesthesia in theatre with the surgeons gowned and ready to start immediately. Use an inhalational induction or minimal dose of methohexitone for induction. Give atropine 0.6 mg IV. Intubate under suxamethonium, taking care to prevent coughing and straining. Maintain anaesthesia with pancuronium, nitrous oxide and phenoperidine. Make sure that the patient is overtransfused by at least 1 litre before the aortic cross-clamp is removed. If hypotension occurs despite adequate transfusion, give digitalis or a dopamine infusion (see Appendix 3). Monitor urine output. Consider postoperative ventilation.

Aneurysm, ruptured aortic. The technique is similar to that described for a leaking aortic *aneurysm*. If the patient is severely shocked, awake intubation is often possible. There is no point trying to replace blood loss or restore the blood pressure until the aorta is clamped.

Aneurysm, thoracic aortic, requires special techniques—e.g. cardiopulmonary bypass. Ask for the assistance of your senior colleagues.

Angiokeratoma corporis diffusum. See *Fabry's disease.*

Angio-osteohypertrophy. See *Klippel–Trenaunay syndrome.*

Anhidrotic ectodermal dysplasia. Maxillofacial abnormalities may hinder intubation. Avoid overheating the patient because sweat glands are absent. Chest infections are common.

Ankylosing spondylitis. These patients may have *restrictive lung disease, aortic regurgitation* and conduction defects. Intubation may be extremely difficult. Therapy may cause anaemia.

Anorexia nervosa. These patients may be hypotensive, hypothermic, anaemic, bradycardic and have electrolyte abnormalities. They may have a *cardiomyopathy* and be sensitive to overtransfusion. Suxamethonium may be potentiated.

Aortic arch syndrome may cause cerebral hypoxia, *renal impairment* and *ischaemic heart disease.* Treatment includes *steroids* and anticoagulants. Use the ECG, CVP, urine output and venous filling to monitor the cardiovascular status, as peripheral pulses are often impalpable.

Aortic regurgitation is often associated with *hypertension.* Avoid hypotension and bradycardia. Err on the side of hypertension and tachycardia but remember that excessive hypertension may precipitate congestive cardiac failure. Antibiotic cover is required.

Aortic stenosis is associated with *ischaemic heart disease* and dysrhythmias. The cardiac output is fixed and the circulation time is slow. During anaesthesia it is important to maintain a normal pulse rate and BP. Dysrhythmias may cause hypotension and should be treated promptly. Antibiotic cover is required.

Apert's syndrome. See *Acrocephalosyndactyly.*

Appendicitis. Check the serum electrolytes preoperatively. Vomiting is rarely severe enough to cause dehydration or electrolyte abnormalities.

Arnold–Chiari syndrome may be associated with *syringomyelia*. During intubation avoid flexion of the neck.

Arsenic poisoning, chronic. Cancers may form at sites of trauma. Antisialogogues are contraindicated. Lubricate the endotracheal tube with water-soluble jelly and intubate atraumatically. Use the minimum number of injection sites.

Arthrogryposis multiplex is sometimes associated with congenital heart disease. Intubation and maintenance of the airway may be difficult. Use respiratory-depressant drugs and muscle relaxants with caution because muscle tone is poor.

Asbestosis. Manage as described for *Pneumoconiosis.*

Ascites may splint the diaphragm and impair ventilation. Associated diseases include *congestive cardiac failure, hepatic impairment* and intra-abdominal malignancy.

Asthma. For severe cases, preoperative physiotherapy, bronchodilators and steroids may help to relieve bronchospasm. Unless there are contraindications, all cases should be given an antihistamine (e.g. chorpheniramine 10 mg IM) and a bronchodilator (e.g. terbutaline 0.25 mg SC) preoperatively. *Steroid* cover may be required. Induce anaesthesia with etomidate and spray the cords with 4% lignocaine. Maintain with nitrous oxide and halothane. Pancuronium is the non-depolarizing muscle relaxant of choice. Thiopentone, tubocurarine and beta-blockers are contraindicated for asthmatics. Postoperatively, give humidified oxygen, keep the patient well hydrated and use narcotic analgesics cautiously if the patient is wheezy. Give nebulized bronchodilators if required.

Atherosclerosis may be associated with *hypertension, obesity, diabetes mellitus, ischaemic heart disease, renal impairment* and *cerebrovascular accidents.* Prevent hypoxia and hypotension, which may increase organ damage.

Atrial ectopic beats. Treatment is not required. Monitor the ECG, however, as atrial ectopic beats may precede the onset of *atrial fibrillation.*

Atrial fibrillation. Preoperative treatment with digitalis or a beta-blocker is required if the peripheral pulse rate is greater than 100 beats per minute or there is a big pulse deficit. Atrial fibrillation of recent onset may revert to sinus rhythm following a DC shock. Atrial fibrillation may be associated with *hyperthyroidism* or heart disease. Pancuronium is contraindicated.

Atrial flutter should be treated preoperatively with digitalis or a DC shock. This dysrhythmia is always associated with heart disease.

Atrial septal defect. Antibiotic cover is required. The uptake of inhalational agents is increased and the effect of intravenous agents is reduced. It is particularly important to give an adequate dose of suxamethonium to ensure good intubating conditions. Prevent hypoxia and hypotension.

Bagassosis. See *Alveolitis, allergic.*

Baló's disease. See *Multiple sclerosis.*

Batten-Turner disease. See *Dystrophia myotonica.*

Beckwith's syndrome. There may be difficulty maintaining the airway or with intubation. Hypoglycaemia is a problem, especially in the neonatal period.

Behçet's syndrome. *Steroids* are used for treatment. Oral scarring may make intubation difficult. Skin pyodermas are common and may make local anaesthesia, especially spinal and epidural anaesthesia, impossible.

Beri-beri is associated with high output cardiac failure and muscle weakness. Use muscle relaxants and respiratory-depressant drugs with care. Thiamine 50–100 mg IV will result in improvement within a few hours.

Berylliosis. Manage as described for *Pneumoconiosis.*

Besnier's fever. See *Sarcoidosis.*

Beta thalassaemia. See *Thalassaemia major* and *minor.*

Bird fancier's lung. See *Alveolitis, allergic.*

Blackfan–Diamond syndrome. Treatment includes blood transfusion and *steroids.*

Bleomycin therapy. These patients may have pulmonary fibrosis but their lung function is usually normal. Never allow the inspired oxygen concentration to rise above 25%. Replace fluids meticulously with colloid rather than crystalloid solutions.

Blind loop syndrome. Anaemia and electrolyte deficiencies may require preoperative correction.

Blindness. Remember that the patient cannot see what is happening. Talk to him throughout induction and any other procedures, particularly if pain may occur.

Bloch–Sulzberger syndrome. See *Incontinentia pigmenti.*

Boeck's fever. See *Sarcoidosis.*

Bourneville's disease. See *Tuberous sclerosis.*

Bowen's syndrome. Polycystic kidneys may cause *renal failure.* Bleeding may occur at operation due to low levels of prothrombin.

Branched-chain ketonuria. A normal anaesthetic may be given. Monitor the blood sugar and blood gases, as hypoglycaemia and metabolic acidosis may occur.

Bronchiectasis. Postural drainage, physiotherapy and antibiotics are of benefit preoperatively. During the operation, oxygenate the patient adequately. Use local anaesthesia if possible.

Bronchiolitis fibrosa obliterans. These patients may require an increased concentration of oxygen and high pressures for inflation of the chest. *Steroids* are used for treatment.

Bronchitis, acute, may progress to *pneumonia* and is an indication for local anaesthesia. If a general anaesthetic is given, pre- and postoperative physiotherapy is useful. Bronchospasm may require treatment. If the causative organism's sensitivity is known, antibiotics should be given.

Bronchitis, chronic, is an indication for local anaesthesia. If a general anaesthetic is given, use IPPV. Use the minimum concentration of oxygen compatible with adequate oxygenation. High concentrations of oxygen may abolish the hypoxic drive to respiration. Bronchospasm and *congestive cardiac failure* may occur. Pre- and postoperative physiotherapy is helpful. Antibiotics should only be given if an organism has been cultured. Beta-blockers are contraindicated.

Budd–Chiari syndrome may be associated with *polycythaemia*, constrictive *pericarditis* or *congestive cardiac failure. Hepatic failure* or *cirrhosis* develop fairly rapidly.

Buerger's disease may be associated with chronic *bronchitis* and *emphysema. Steroids* and vasodilators are used for treatment. Prevent trauma to the extremities and use local anaesthesia if possible. The patient may be sensitive to fluid loss.

Bulbar palsy is associated with *motor neuron disease* and recurrent chest infections secondary to aspiration.

Bundle branch block, combined left and right. These patients may require temporary pacing. A cardiologist should be consulted.

Bundle branch block, left. No treatment is required.

Bundle branch block, right. No treatment is required.

Burkitt's lymphoma. Intubation may be difficult.

Burns. If the burn is greater than 15% (1 patient's hand = 1%), the patient will lose large volumes of fluid in the first 48 hours after the burn. This should be replaced with plasma or dextran 110 supplemented by blood. Monitor the pulse rate, BP, CVP, packed cell volume and urine output as a guide to the adequacy of fluid replacement. Inhalation of smoke may cause laryngeal and pulmonary oedema, bronchospasm and carbon monoxide poisoning, which should be treated with high concentrations of oxygen. During anaesthesia be prepared for a difficult intubation due to swelling or scarring, and massive blood loss which may be reduced by a hypotensive technique. Use a warming blanket and warm fluids. Suxamethonium is contraindicated from 15 to 66 days after the burn.

Byssinosis. Manage as described for *Pneumoconiosis.*

Caplan's syndrome consists of *rheumatoid arthritis*, rounded opacities and pulmonary fibrosis in a miner.

Carcinoid syndrome. Ideally the patient should be given cyproheptadine 4 mg orally 8-hourly for 24 hours preoperatively. Premedicate the patient with chlorpromazine 20–50 mg IM. Induce with thiopentone. Suxamethonium should be avoided if possible, as it may cause hypotension. Maintain anaesthesia with nitrous oxide, fentanyl and droperidol (5–10 mg). Use pancuronium for muscle relaxation. Treat *hypertension* with methotrimeprazine 2.5–5.0 mg increments IV. Treat hypotension with an aprotinin infusion given at 200000 units per hour. Aprotinin may be diluted in physiological saline solution. Methoxamine also may be used for hypotension. Bronchospasm should be treated with aprotinin. It has been recommended that methylprednisolone 1 g IV 6-hourly be given for 24 hours. During anaesthesia prevent hypotension, hypoxia and acidosis. Morphine, tubocurarine, ephedrine, noradrenaline and metaraminol are contraindicated. *Pulmonary stenosis* and *tricuspid stenosis* are associated with carcinoid syndrome.

Cardiac tamponade. Pericardiocentesis should be performed under local anaesthesia. The patient should then be anaesthetized using minimal concentrations of inhalational agents. IPPV should only be used after the pleura has been opened. An isoprenaline infusion (see Appendix 3) may be helpful until the pericardium has been opened.

Cardio-auditory syndrome. See *Jervell–Nielsen syndrome.*

Cardiomyopathy, congestive. These patients have severe *congestive cardiac failure.* They rarely survive any form of surgery. Dysrhythmias are common. Atropine should be given at induction. Use minimal doses of other drugs, and avoid hypoxia, bradycardia and hypotension. Halothane is contraindicated.

Cardiomyopathy, hypertrophic, is treated with beta-blockers, digitalis and diuretics. These patients are severely ill and should be anaesthetized by the method described for congestive *cardiomyopathy.* Halothane and catecholamines are contraindicated.

Carotid artery occlusion, acute, is treated by carotid endarterectomy. *Atherosclerosis* may affect other organs.

Carpenter's syndrome may be associated with congenital heart disease. Intubation may be difficult.

Cerebral abscess. May cause raised *intracranial pressure*.

Cerebral gigantism. See *Sotos' syndrome*.

Cerebrovascular accident may be due to haemorrhage, embolism or thrombosis. Look for evidence of myocardial disease. While muscle wasting is proceeding rapidly in the first few weeks after a cerebrovascular accident, suxamethonium is contraindicated. During anaesthesia prevent hypoxia, hypotension and hypertension. Maintain normocarbia.

Cervical spondylitis. Intubation may be difficult.

Chagas' disease. See *Trypanosomiasis, American*.

Charcot-Marie-Tooth disease. See *Motor neuron disease, lower*.

Chédiak-Higashi syndrome. The platelet count may be low. Use aseptic techniques. *Steroids* may be used for treatment.

Cherubism. Multiple tumours of the jaw and soft tissues of the mouth may make intubation difficult. A tracheostomy performed under local anaesthesia may be necessary to relieve severe respiratory distress.

Chondroectodermal dysplasia. See *Ellis-van Creveld syndrome*.

Chondro-osteodystrophy. See *Morquio's syndrome*.

Chotzen syndrome. *Renal impairment* or *failure* may occur. Intubation is difficult.

Christmas disease. Give factor IX concentrate according to the advice of a haematologist.

Chronic granulomatous disease. Pulmonary function is often poor. Use local anaesthesia if possible. Maintain strict asepsis to prevent infection.

Chronic non-suppurative panniculitis. See *Weber-Christian disease*.

Cigarette smoking is associated with chronic *bronchitis*, *ischaemic heart disease* and *peripheral vascular disease*. Dysrhythmias may occur with adrenaline and aminophylline.

Cirrhosis. A spectrum of conditions ranging from mild disturbance of liver function to *hepatic failure* may occur. Check clotting factors, haemoglobin, electrolytes and blood sugar preoperatively. Do not pass a nasogastric tube if oesophageal varices may be present. Premedicate with diazepam or pethidine unless the patient has gross hepatic failure. Induce anaesthesia with Althesin or thiopentone. Maintain anaesthesia with nitrous oxide and small doses of fentanyl or pethidine, and muscle relaxation with pancuronium.

Clotting factor antibodies. Uncontrollable bleeding may occur. Treatment is often unsuccessful but *steroids* and exchange transfusion may help.

Coarctation of the aorta. Give antibiotic cover. Hypertension occurs in the upper half of the body. The blood pressure may be higher in the right arm than in the left. During anaesthesia prevent hypoxia, hypertension and hypotension. If the chest is being operated on, be prepared for excessive blood loss from the collateral circulation.

Coma, hepatic. See *Hepatic failure.* Sedative drugs and narcotic analgesics are contraindicated.

Congenital anhidrotic ectodermal defect. The airway may be difficult to maintain and intubation is difficult. Avoid overheating the patient because sweat glands are absent. Tape the eyes shut because tears are not formed. Give humidified oxygen and physiotherapy postoperatively.

Congenital facial diplegia. See *Möbius' syndrome.*

Congenital fibrinogen deficiency. Give fibrinogen as advised by a haematologist.

Congestive cardiac failure. The condition of the patient may be improved preoperatively by bed rest, a low-sodium diet, correction of electrolyte abnormalities, diuretics and digitalis. The patient should be sitting on the journey to theatre and during induction. During anaesthesia, use IPPV and prevent hypoxia and hypercarbia. Transfuse fluids cautiously to prevent overload.

Conn's syndrome. See *Aldosteronism, primary.*

Conradi's syndrome consists of *renal impairment* and congenital heart disease.

Cooley's anaemia. See *Thalassaemia.*

Cor pulmonale. Treat infection, bronchospasm and pulmonary oedema if necessary. These patients should only be digitalized if dysrhythmias are present.

Coryza. Postoperative physiotherapy may help to prevent infection of the lower respiratory tract. Use local anaesthesia if possible.

Cranial arteritis is treated with *steroids.* Avoid hypotension, which may cause blindness. Watch for pharyngeal oedema postoperatively, which may obstruct the airway and sometimes

occurs in association with cranial arteritis.

Cretinism is congenital hypothyroidism. Intubation may be difficult. Preoperatively, check serum electrolytes and blood sugar because cretins are prone to hyponatraemia and hypoglycaemia. These patients are extremely sensitive to respiratory-depressant drugs. They have a low cardiac output and tolerate hypovolaemia poorly. Transfuse with caution because overload may precipitate cardiac failure. During the operation prevent hypoxia and hypotension.

Cri-du-chat syndrome. Laryngomalacia may cause difficulty in maintaining the airway and intubation.

Crist–Siemens–Touraine syndrome. See *Anhidrotic ectodermal dysplasia*.

Crohn's disease. *Steroids* form part of the treatment. Dehydration, electrolyte deficiencies and protein deficiency should be corrected preoperatively.

Crouzon's disease. These patients are *obese*. Craniofacial dysostosis and a stiff neck may make intubation difficult. Nasal intubation may be impossible due to nasal obstruction.

Cushing's disease is managed in the same way as *Cushing's syndrome*.

Cushing's syndrome is associated with *diabetes mellitus*, *hypertension*, *obesity*, osteoporosis and *congestive cardiac failure*. The electrolytes should be checked and abnormalities corrected preoperatively, particularly hypokalaemia which may be severe. *Steroid* cover should be given. Aseptic techniques are necessary to prevent infection. Bearing in mind the associated diseases, use IPPV and prevent hypotension, hypertension and hypoxia. Thiopentone, pancuronium and fentanyl have been suggested as suitable drugs. The skin and bones are fragile, so the patient should be moved with care.

Cutis laxa. These patients are prone to chronic *bronchitis*, *emphysema* and *cor pulmonale*. Lax tissues may cause laryngeal obstruction and difficulty in maintaining drip sites.

Cyclic neutropenia. *Steroid* cover and antibiotics should be given.

Cystic fibrosis involves the lungs, pancreas and liver. The patient may have *cirrhosis* or *diabetes mellitus*. Treatment of the lungs includes antibiotics, postural drainage and physiotherapy. Premedicate with diazepam. Atropine is contraindicated. An inhalational induction combined with suxamethonium has been suggested. Ventilate the patient, maintaining relaxation with small doses of muscle relaxant, and anaesthesia with humidified nitrous oxide and halothane given with 50% oxygen. Postural drainage and physiotherapy should be given before the patient is extubated. Postoperatively, continue postural drainage and physiotherapy. Give humidified oxygen.

Cystinuria. These patients may get renal stones, which cause *renal failure*. Prevent dehydration and maintain a good urine output to prevent stone formation.

Deafness. These patients should be allowed to wear a hearing aid until anaesthesia has been induced. Remember to position yourself so that the patient can lip read when you are talking to him.

Deep vein thrombosis. These patients may be taking anticoagulants. If there is a history of deep vein thrombosis, consider using anti-embolism stockings, subcutaneous heparin or a dextran 70 infusion. Support the ankles to prevent pressure on the calves.

Degos' syndrome. All organs may be affected by arteriolar thrombosis. Bowel involvement causes hypoproteinaemia, which may alter drug binding. Oral scarring may hamper intubation.

Déjérine–Sottas disease. See *Motor neuron disease, lower.*

Dermatomyositis may be associated with *myasthenic syndrome, hepatic impairment, myocarditis, scleroderma* and *steroid therapy.*

Detached retina. See p. 162 for the anaesthetic management.

Devic's disease. See *Multiple sclerosis.*

Dextrocardia. Isolated dextrocardia is usually associated with other cardiac abnormalities. If all the organs are reversed, the heart is usually normal.

Diabetes insipidus, if untreated, leads to severe electrolyte deficiencies and dehydration, which should be corrected preoperatively.

Diabetes mellitus (on oral hypoglycaemics). Check the blood sugar preoperatively. If it is less than 4.4 mmol/l, give 50% dextrose 25 ml IV. Give all cases 5% dextrose 100 ml per hour peroperatively. Postoperatively check the blood sugar. Some patients may require soluble insulin. If the blood sugar is normal, continue 5% dextrose 100 ml per hour until the patient is able to resume his normal diet.

Diabetes mellitus (on insulin). Associated conditions include *ischaemic heart disease, cerebrovascular accidents* and autonomic *neuropathy*. All patients should have their blood sugar checked preoperatively.

Controlled diabetics: major operation. If the patient has had his morning dose of insulin, give 50% dextrose 25–50 ml IV. All patients should be given 5% dextrose 2 litres peroperatively with soluble insulin 10–15 units in each litre. Monitor the blood sugar and alter the dose of insulin according to the results. During anaesthesia avoid hypoxia, hypercarbia, propranolol and ganglion-blocking agents. Postoperatively, monitor the blood sugar levels with reagent sticks. Send a sample to the laboratory periodically to check the accuracy of the sticks. Maintain the blood sugar at 6–10 mmol with an insulin infusion. Usually 2–4 units per hour is required. Give prochlorperazine 12.5 mg IM 6-hourly as required to prevent vomiting.

Controlled diabetics: minor operations. Preoperatively, the management is the same as for major operations. As the operation is brief, blood sugar monitoring is unnecessary. Postoperatively, measure the blood sugar. If it is normal, give 5% dextrose 100 ml per hour until the patient is eating normally. Resumption of eating should be encouraged as soon as the patient will tolerate it. If the blood sugar is more than 15 mmol/l, give insulin and treat the patient as if he has had a major operation.

Uncontrolled diabetics. These patients should be controlled preoperatively. A suitable regimen is:

(1) Pass a nasogastric tube and leave it to drain freely.
(2) Fluids: physiological saline solution 1 litre in ½ hour;
     physiological saline solution 1 litre in 1 hour;
     physiological saline solution 1 litre in 2 hours;
     then physiological saline solution 500 ml 4-hourly

Monitor the blood sugar hourly and follow the above regimen until the blood sugar is less than 14 mmol/l. Then give 5% dextrose 500 ml containing 13 mmol potassium chloride 4-hourly. Give also soluble insulin 8 units SC 4-hourly. Check the adequacy of the regimen by monitoring the blood sugar.

(3) Potassium. In the early stages give potassium chloride 13 mmol per hour. Monitor the serum potassium hourly. If it is less than 4 mmol/l, give 26 mmol per hour in the drip. If it is greater than 6 mmol/l, stop giving potassium. When the blood sugar is less than 14 mmol/l, give potassium chloride as described above.

(4) Acidosis. Maintain the pH at more than 7.1 with sodium bicarbonate (see p. 17).

(5) Hyperosmolar coma. Treat by rehydration with potassium supplements. Only very small doses of insulin should be given. Often none is required.

Diarrhoea. Up to 4 litres of fluid per day may be lost, causing hypovolaemia, hypokalaemia and possibly hypoproteinaemia and metabolic acidosis. Deficits should be corrected preoperatively.

Di George's syndrome is associated with *hypoparathyroidism*, recurrent *bronchitis* and aortic arch abnormalities which restrict the cardiac output. Prevent hypoxia and hypotension.

Di Gugliemo's disease. See *Leukaemia*.

Disseminated intravascular coagulation is caused by septicaemia and obstetric disasters. Treatment should be recommended by a haematologist.

Disseminated sclerosis. See *Multiple sclerosis*.

Diverticular disease. Anaesthetic problems are secondary to severe *diarrhoea* or *intestinal obstruction*.

Down's syndrome is often associated with congenital heart disease. Atropine is contraindicated because fatal idiosyncracies have occurred. Intubation may be difficult. Ensure adequate oxygenation prior to extubation because laryngospasm is common.

Dysautonomia, familial. These patients have a fixed heart rate, labile BP, inability to sweat and insensitivity to pain. Recurrent chest infections are common. Atropine and hyoscine are contraindicated. Chlorpromazine 0.5–1.0 mg/kg IM should be used for premedication. Use thiopentone and halothane with extreme caution and avoid their use if possible. Use IPPV. Supplement with small doses of fentanyl to prevent postoperative respiratory depression. Monitor the BP and temperature closely. Treat hypertension with phenoxybenzamine, and hypotension with fluid and *small* doses of adrenaline (i.e. 0.1 µg/kg per minute). These patients are very sensitive to catecholamines. Use oxygen cautiously because these patients' respiratory centres are insensitive to hypercarbia.

Dystonia musculorum deformans. See *Torsion dystonia*.

Dystrophia myotonica. Avoid respiratory depressant drugs. Narcotic analgesics and diazepam are contraindicated. Use Althesin or very small doses of thiopentone for induction. Then give oxygen with nitrous oxygen and enflurane or trichloroethylene for intubation. Suxamethonium and halothane are contraindicated. Monitor the ECG because dysrhythmias are common. *Congestive cardiac failure* may also occur. Monitor the temperature, as these patients have an increased risk of malignant hyperpyrexia. Small doses of tubocurarine may be used but neostigmine is contraindicated. Spinal and epidural anaesthesia do not prevent myotonia. Spinal anaesthesia may precipitate myotonia. Rarely, adrenal insufficiency occurs. *Steroids* should be given. Postoperatively, do not extubate the patient until the risk of respiratory depression has passed and a good cough reflex is present. If myotonia occurs, try treating it by infiltrating the muscle with local anaesthetic or giving procainamide 100 mg per minute IV up to 600 mg or diphenylhydantoin 300–600 mg IV. Hyperkalaemia and postoperative shivering should be prevented as they may precipitate myotonia.

Ebstein's anomaly. Supraventricular tachycardia is common at induction. Peroperatively, dysrhythmias and congestive cardiac failure may occur. Prevent myocardial depression, hypoxia and hypotension.

Eccentro-osteochondrodysplasia. See *Morquio's syndrome.*

Ehlers–Danlos syndrome. Connective tissue weakness may affect the function of the heart, kidneys, pancreas and liver. The mucous membranes and skin are fragile. There may be difficulty in maintaining intravenous infusions. Intramuscular injections should be avoided. Minor trauma to the respiratory tract may cause bleeding.

Eisenmenger's syndrome. These patients may be taking anticoagulants. Prevent hypoxia and hypotension. Prevent vasodilatation, which may increase the shunt and cause hypoxia. Prevent vasoconstriction, which may decrease the shunt and reduce cardiac output. Use IPPV but check that the patient is adequately reversed. Epidural anaesthesia has been used successfully.

Ellis–van Creveld syndrome. Skeletal abnormalities may cause intubation difficulty and restriction of chest wall movement. Lung function is, therefore, poor.

Embolism, femoral artery. The clot should be removed under local anaesthesia if possible, as these patients have often had a recent myocardial infarction or dysrhythmia. Be prepared, however, to proceed to a laparotomy.

Embolism, pulmonary. The patient may be anticoagulated. Patients requiring surgical removal of the embolism should be ventilated gently with 100% oxygen until the clot is removed.

Ketamine or fentanyl should be used to provide anaesthesia, and pancuronium to provide muscle relaxation. A dopamine infusion (see Appendix 3) may raise the blood pressure. If there is a history of pulmonary embolism, consider giving subcutaneous heparin or dextran 70. The patient should wear anti-embolism stockings and have his ankles supported to prevent pressure on his calves during anaesthesia.

Emphysema. Physiotherapy is of little benefit unless the patient has an acute chest infection. The work of breathing is increased. Severe cases develop *congestive cardiac failure*. Local anaesthesia is preferable. If general anaesthesia is unavoidable, use IPPV.

Empyema. This should be drained under local anaesthesia to allow re-expansion of the lung. If the empyema ruptures into a bronchus, a bronchopleural *fistula* is formed.

Encephalitis. If muscle wasting is occurring, suxamethonium is contraindicated.

Encephalotrigeminal angiomatosis. Also known as *Sturge–Weber syndrome. Epilepsy* is the major problem.

Enchondromatosis. See *Ollier's disease.*

Endocarditis, infective. These patients are prone to *ischaemic heart disease*, dysrhythmias and intractable *congestive cardiac failure*. Antibiotic cover should be given.

Engelmann's disease. Intubation is made difficult by inability to open the mouth and a stiff neck. An inhalational induction and blind nasal intubation may be required.

Epidermolysis bullosa. Prevent trauma to ectodermal tissues. Friction causes more damage than direct pressure. *Steroid* cover is required. Allow the patient to climb onto the table himself. Rest the face mask on muslin soaked in 0.5% hydrocortisone. Induce with intravenous ketamine. If intubation is essential, it should be atraumatic and the tube should be lubricated with hydrocortisone cream. If buccal or palatal bleeding occurs, tilt the patient head down and apply sponges soaked in adrenaline (1:200 000). Use muscle relaxants with caution. If muscle wasting is occurring, suxamethonium may cause hyperkalaemia and fatal dysrhythmias. The action of non-depolarizing relaxants is unpredictable. Local anaesthesia is often unsuitable because of contractures and infection.

NB. *Porphyria* may produce similar lesions and be misdiagnosed as epidermolysis bullosa.

Epilepsy. Maintain anticonvulsant therapy pre- and postoperatively. Methohexitone, propanidid, Althesin, ketamine and enflurane are contraindicated. Prevent hypoxia, hypotension and increased body temperature.

Erythema multiforme. Check fluid and electrolyte balance preoperatively. Give *steroid* cover if necessary. Intubation may be difficult. Postoperative laryngeal oedema may cause airway obstruction.

Erythema nodosum may be associated with *sarcoidosis, tuberculosis* and *ulcerative colitis. Steroids* are sometimes used for treatment.

Erythraemia. See *Polycythaemia, primary.*

Erythrocytosis. See *Polycythaemia.*

Eulenberg syndrome. See *Paramyotonia congenita.*

Extradural haematoma. See *Intracranial pressure, raised.*

Fabry's disease is associated with *ischaemic heart disease, renal impairment, hypertension* and *cerebrovascular accidents.* Oedema of the face may make intubation difficult and oedema of the hands hinders cannulation of veins. Oral telangiectases may bleed if traumatized during intubation.

Factor V deficiency. Treat preoperatively with fresh-frozen plasma.

Factor VII deficiency. This is not usually a problem. If bleeding is difficult to control, give fresh-frozen plasma.

Factor VIII deficiency. See *Haemophilia.*

Factor IX deficiency. See *Christmas disease.*

Factor XII deficiency may increase the partial thromboplastin time but does not cause bleeding.

Factor XIII deficiency may be corrected by blood transfusion. It does not usually cause significant bleeding.

Fallot's tetralogy. Antibiotic cover is required. Before surgical correction beta-blockers are used to control cyanotic attacks. Use minimal doses of induction agents and IPPV. Maintain a normal blood pressure and prevent hypoxia.

Familial periodic paralysis, hyperkalaemic. Attacks are precipitated by exercise and cold. The respiratory muscles are not affected. During preoperative starvation, give a 5% dextrose infusion. An attack should be treated with glucose and insulin, or adrenaline. During the operation keep the patient warm. Muscle relaxants are contraindicated.

Familial periodic paralysis, hypokalaemic. Attacks are precipitated by glucose, insulin, adrenaline, steroids, trauma, menstruation, stress and infection. Sodium and water retention may cause *congestive cardiac failure.* Give a sedative premedicant and use a normal anaesthetic technique. Avoid giving large volumes of 5% dextrose. Treat an attack with 10–100 mmol potassium chloride given in an infusion. During an attack the patient is resistant to suxamethonium and sensitive to non-depolarizing relaxants. The patient should be nursed in an intensive care unit postoperatively, as stress may precipitate an attack several hours after the operation is over.

Familial periodic paralysis, normokalaemic. Attacks are precipitated by the same factors as the hypokalaemic type except for glucose. Hyperkalaemia also provokes attacks. Give a normal anaesthetic. Ventricular extrasystoles may occur and should be treated with lignocaine.

Familial xanthomatosis. See *Wolman's disease.*

Fanconi syndrome. See *Acidosis, renal tubular.*

Farber's disease is associated with *congestive cardiac failure* and *renal failure.* Intubation may be difficult due to laryngeal deposits.

Farmer's lung. See *Alveolitis, allergic.*

Favism. See *Glucose-6-phosphate dehydrogenase deficiency.*

Felty's syndrome. *Rheumatoid arthritis* is part of the syndrome. *Steroids* may be used for treatment.

Fibrinogenopenia. Give cryoprecipitate preoperatively. A haematologist should be consulted.

Fibrodysplasia ossificans. Chest wall restriction may cause pulmonary insufficiency. *Steroids* may be used for treatment. Intubation may be difficult due to inability to open the mouth and a stiff neck. Use local anaesthesia if possible.

Fistula, biliary. About 1500 ml per day may be lost, causing electrolyte deficiencies and metabolic acidosis. These abnormalities should be corrected preoperatively.

Fistula, bronchopleural. The patient should be brought to theatre and anaesthetized sitting upright but tilted laterally so that the damaged side is inferior. A chest drain should be inserted before anaesthesia is induced. IPPV should not be used until a double-lumen endobronchial tube has been passed and the good lung isolated from the bad lung. If the leak from the damaged lung is large, it may be necessary to ventilate only the good lung and insufflate oxygen into the damaged lung.

Fistula, distal small bowel and colonic. Losses are usually less than 1500 ml per day. Dehydration and electrolyte deficiencies are uncommon.

Fistula, duodenal. These patients may lose up to 7 litres per day. Severe dehydration and electrolyte deficiency should be corrected preoperatively.

Fistula, gastric. Up to 7 litres per day may be lost, causing severe dehydration and electrolyte deficiency. Deficits should be corrected preoperatively.

Fistula, high small bowel. Losses of up to 5 litres per day should be replaced with physiological saline solution.

Fistula, pulmonary arteriovenous. Cyanosis is not improved by oxygen. There may be secondary *polycythaemia*. Maintain good oxygenation throughout anaesthesia.

Focal dermal hypoplasia. See *Gorlin–Goltz syndrome*.

Forbes' disease may be associated with *congestive cardiac failure*. Hypoglycaemia may occur during anaesthesia. The blood sugar should be monitored.

Fractured femur may be secondary to a blackout caused by myocardial or cerebral disease. The patient may have lost up to 2 litres of blood. Resuscitation should be done preoperatively. Consider a unilateral spinal if there is no evidence of heart disease.

Fragilitas osseum. See *Osteogenesis imperfecta*.

Friedreich's ataxia causes combined upper and lower *motor neuron disease*. Scoliosis may cause respiratory insufficiency. *Congestive cardiac failure* and *diabetes mellitus* also occur.

Fructosaemia is associated with *renal* and *hepatic impairment*. Hypoglycaemic episodes and transient bleeding diatheses may occur. These patients should be managed by the same method as that described for *galactosaemia*.

Gaisböck's disease consists of primary *polycythaemia* and *hypertension*.

Galactosaemia. Give 50% dextrose 25 ml at induction and monitor the blood sugar throughout. *Hepatic impairment* and *renal failure* occur late in the disease.

Ganglioneuroma may secrete vasoactive hormones. Management is the same as that described for *phaeochromocytoma*.

Gardner's syndrome consists of multiple tumours of soft tissue, bone and the intestine. Intubation may be very difficult. Repeat operations are often required, and a tracheostomy performed early may be an advantage. It may also be required to relieve airway obstruction.

Gastrectomy. Anaemia and persistent *diarrhoea* may be present many years after the operation.

Gaucher's disease. Usually there are no anaesthetic problems. Bulbar palsy may lead to aspiration and recurrent chest infections. Bleeding problems are sometimes associated with platelet deficiency.

Giant cell arteritis. See *Cranial arteritis*.

Glanzmann's disease. See *Thrombasthenia*.

Glaucoma. Acute-angle glaucoma is precipitated by atropine and mydriatics. Atropine 0.006 mg/kg IM is safe. Open-angle glaucoma is precipitated by steroids. Suxamethonium may be used, as it causes only a brief rise in intraocular pressure.

Glomerulonephritis, acute. *Steroids* are used for treatment. *Hypertension* and *left ventricular failure* may occur.

Glomerulonephritis, chronic, sometimes follows an acute episode and may progress to *renal failure*.

Glucose-6-phosphate dehydrogenase deficiency. Haemolysis may be precipitated by prilocaine, acetylsalicylic acid, paracetamol, sulphonamides, chloramphenicol, quinidine and methylene blue. These drugs should be avoided. During an attack treat anaemia with packed red cells. Maintain a good urine output at all times.

Glycogen storage disease, type I. See *von Gierke's disease*.

Glycogen storage disease, type II. See *Pompe's disease*.

Glycogen storage disease, type III. See *Forbes' disease*.

Glycogen storage disease, type IV. See *Andersen's disease*.

Glycogen storage disease, type V. See *McArdle's disease*.

Glycogen storage disease, type VI. See *Hers' disease*.

Glycogen storage disease, type VII. See *McArdle's disease*.

Glycogen synthetase deficiency. Hypoglycaemia may occur. Monitor the blood sugar and give 50% dextrose 25 ml IV as required. Use a 5% dextrose infusion peroperatively.

Goldenhar's syndrome. Facial abnormalities may make intubation difficult. There often is associated congenital heart disease.

Goodpasture's syndrome is associated with *glomerulonephritis*. Severe haemorrhage may occur into one lung, which should be isolated using a Robertshaw tube. *Steroids* are used for treatment.

Gorlin–Goltz syndrome. Asymmetry of the head may make intubation difficult. There may be congenital heart disease and renal anomalies.

Gout is associated with cricoarytenoid arthritis and *ischaemic heart disease*. Gout may be precipitated by anxiety and a poor urine output, lactate solutions and methoxyflurane. Give a sedative premedicant. Prepare for a difficult intubation. Maintain a good urine output with 5% dextrose solution or physiological saline solution.

Graves' disease. See *Hyperthyroidism.*

Groenblad–Strandberg syndrome is associated with *hypertension, ischaemic heart disease* and *cerebrovascular accidents.* Functioning intravenous cannulae may be difficult to maintain.

Guillain–Barré syndrome. The autonomic nervous system is disturbed. To prevent hypotension, change the patient's posture slowly, replace blood loss promptly, ventilate with the minimum effective intrathoracic pressure and give barbiturates cautiously. Preload with fluid before giving a spinal anaesthetic. Monitor the ECG because dysrhythmias are common. Suxamethonium is contraindicated for at least 3 months after the onset of the illness. *Steroids* are sometimes used for treatment.

Haematemesis usually implies a large bleed from the upper gastrointestinal tract. An attempt should be made to replace the losses preoperatively. Full resuscitation may not be possible in the presence of torrential active bleeding. An attempt should be made to empty the stomach prior to induction. NB. Blind passage of a nasogastric tube is contraindicated if oesophageal varices are present. However, an experienced physician may be able to pass a Sengstaken tube and stop variceal bleeding.

Haemochromatosis may cause *cirrhosis, renal impairment* and *diabetes mellitus.* Myocardial involvement causes dysrhythmias and *congestive cardiac failure.*

Haemoglobin C thalassaemia. Anaemia is mild. Usually there are no anaesthetic problems.

Haemoglobin H. Sulphonamides are contraindicated. There are no anaesthetic problems.

Haemoglobin M. Methaemoglobinaemia, for which there is no treatment, causes cyanosis and reduced oxygen-carrying capacity of the blood. Give at least 30% oxygen during and after the operation. Prilocaine is contraindicated.

Haemophilia. Give factor VIII concentrate to raise serum levels to 35% of normal. Avoid intramuscular injections. Spinal and epidural anaesthesia are contraindicated. Intubate atraumatically. Nasal intubation is contraindicated.

Haemorrhage, post-adenoidectomy. If possible, the post-nasal space should be packed without anaesthesia. If anaesthesia is essential, pass a nasogastric tube and empty the stomach. Correct blood loss preoperatively. Use an inhalational induction in the head-down position if haemorrhage may obscure the airway.

Haemorrhage, post-thyroidectomy. Open the wound and evacuate the clot without anaesthesia. If this is impossible, do an awake intubation with or without anaesthesia.

Haemorrhage, post-tonsillectomy. Use a technique similar to that described for post-adenoidectomy *haemorrhage*.

Haemosiderosis. The problems are similar to those for *haemochromatosis*.

Hamman–Rich syndrome. *Steroids* are used for treatment. Oxygen and anaesthetic gases diffuse poorly across the alveolar membrane. In severe cases, total intravenous anaesthesia may have to be given. *Congestive heart failure* may occur. High concentrations of oxygen should be given if necessary to prevent hypoxia.

Hand–Schüller–Christian disease. *Steroid* cover is required. *Hepatic impairment* and *diabetes insipidus* may occur. Bone marrow involvement causes anaemia, platelet deficiency and increased susceptibility to infection. Laryngeal fibrosis may make intubation difficult. Pulmonary fibrosis leads to *cor pulmonale*. The teeth may be loose.

Hashimoto's thyroiditis. These patients may be euthyroid or *hypothyroid*.

Heart block, complete. The patient should have a temporary pacemaker inserted preoperatively. If this is not possible, use an isoprenaline infusion to increase the heart rate to 50 beats per minute. Prevent hypoxia, hypotension and hypovolaemia peroperatively. Note that tachycardia does not occur in response to inadequate anaesthesia.

Heart block, first-degree, may be a sign of digitalis toxicity or a recent myocardial infarction. No treatment is required unless the rate is less than 50 beats per minute, when atropine 0.6 mg IV should be given at induction.

Heart block, second-degree. Treat with atropine 0.6 mg IV preoperatively. Have a temporary pacing wire and box available in the theatre, as second-degree heart block sometimes progresses to complete heart block.

Heart–hand syndrome. See *Holt–Oram syndrome*.

Heavy gamma chain disease. These patients may be anaemic and are prone to infection. Use aseptic techniques. *Steroid* cover may be required.

Henoch–Schönlein purpura. Rarely, these patients develop *renal failure*.

Hepatic failure. The signs include encephalopathy, *jaundice*, haemorrhage, hypotension, tachycardia and *renal failure*. The prothrombin time is prolonged. Preoperatively, check and correct abnormalities of the serum electrolytes and blood glucose. Give fresh-frozen plasma, platelets and whole blood to correct the clotting abnormality and blood loss. Give 10% calcium gluconate 10 ml with each litre of blood. Induce anaesthesia with diazepam 5 mg or very small quantities of thiopentone if the patient is conscious. Intubate using suxamethonium. Ventilate with nitrous oxide and oxygen, using pancuronium for muscle relaxation. Narcotic analgesics may aggravate hepatic coma. Use low concentrations of trichloroethylene or halothane to supplement anaesthesia if necessary. Give 5% dextrose solution to replace insensible losses.

Hepatic impairment may range from abnormal liver function tests, which usually cause no problem to the anaesthetist, to overt *hepatic failure*. Always check the clotting factors and correct abnormalities preoperatively. Use sedatives and narcotic analgesics with caution, as their action may be prolonged. Pancuronium is the non-depolarizing muscle relaxant of choice.

Hepatitis. All cases have *hepatic impairment*. Patients with hepatitis B need special precautions so that theatre personnel do not become infected. Infection is transmitted via the patient's blood and secretions. Only the minimum number of people should attend to the patient. Use disposable equipment whenever possible. Wear a gown, gloves and a mask. Clean up spilled blood with a hypochlorite–detergent solution. Each hospital will have its own protocol for the sterilization of non-disposable equipment.

Hepatolenticular degeneration. See *Kinnier Wilson's disease*.

Hereditary angioneurotic oedema. Give fresh-frozen plasma 6 packs at least 40 minutes preoperatively. Intubate as gently as possible. All trauma may cause oedema. This may cause respiratory obstruction if it occurs in the face or larynx. Following extubation, watch the patient closely for signs of respiratory obstruction. Reintubation may be necessary. Treat an attack with fresh-frozen plasma, adrenaline 0.5 mg SC and an antihistamine.

Hereditary atactica polyneuritis. See *Refsum's disease*.

Hereditary elliptocytosis. These patients may require preoperative blood transfusion to correct anaemia.

Hereditary haemorrhagic telangiectasia. Avoid trauma to the skin and mucous membranes, as haemorrhage may occur. Telangiectases in the lungs may cause high-output cardiac failure, or haemorrhage into a lung which may have to be isolated with a Robertshaw tube. Preoperative blood transfusion may be required to correct anaemia due to chronic blood loss. Recurrent chest infections are common. Give postoperative physiotherapy.

Hereditary spherocytosis. *Steroids* are sometimes used for treatment. Anaemia may require correction preoperatively.

Hermanski–Pudlak syndrome. See *Chédiak–Higashi syndrome*.

Hernia, diaphragmatic. Bowel in the thorax may compress the lung, causing hypoxia and problems similar to those of *restrictive lung disease*.

Hernia, hiatus, is associated with an increased risk of regurgitation.

Hernia, Richter's. Part of the bowel wall is strangulated. Intestinal obstruction does not occur but part of the bowel may have to be resected. Spinal anaesthesia is contraindicated.

Hernia, strangulated. Vomiting and intestinal obstruction occur. Dehydration, electrolyte deficiencies and hypoproteinaemia should be corrected preoperatively.

Hers' disease. Hypoglycaemia may occur. Give 5% dextrose solution peroperatively and monitor the blood sugar.

Histiocytosis X. See *Hand–Schüller–Christian disease*.

Hoffman's disease. See *Dystrophia myotonica*.

Holt–Oram syndrome is associated with congenital heart disease.

Homocystinuria. These patients are prone to thrombosis. Prevent dehydration, hypotension and venous pooling. Use anti-embolism stockings, support the ankles to relieve pressure on the calves and consider subcutaneous heparin or an infusion of dextran 70.

Hunter's syndrome. The larynx may be involved and cause intubation difficulty. *Pneumonia* and *congestive cardiac failure* may occur.

Huntington's chorea. Thiopentone may cause spasm of the jaws and delayed awakening. Small doses have been used safely but an inhalation induction is probably better. These patients may be sensitive to suxamethonium and non-depolarizing relaxants which should be used in small doses.

Hurler's syndrome. Intubation may be difficult. Abnormal tracheobronchial cartilages may cause partial collapse of the airways and frequent respiratory infections. *Ischaemic heart disease* and *congestive cardiac failure* may occur. Preoperative physiotherapy may be of benefit. Use an inhalational induction for intubation. Avoid dehydration. Postoperatively, give humidified oxygen.

Hutchinson–Gilford syndrome. See *Progeria.*

Hydatid disease. Cysts may reduce the function of the lungs, heart, brain, kidney and liver. Anaphylactic shock may occur if the cyst ruptures as it is removed.

Hydatidiform mole. Thyrotropin secretion may cause severe *hyperthyroidism.*

Hydronephrosis. *Renal failure* may occur.

Hyperbetalipoproteinaemia causes *ischaemic heart disease* and *peripheral vascular disease.*

Hyperinsulinism. Recurrent hypoglycaemia occurs. Give 50% dextrose 25–50 ml to cover the starvation period. The anaesthetic technique is not important except that volatile agents should be avoided. Monitor the blood sugar frequently. An infusion of 10% dextrose may be required to maintain the blood sugar. It should be given through a central vein.

Hyperoxaluria. Maintain a good urine output to prevent precipitation of oxalate crystals which may cause *renal failure.* Prevent hypotension.

Hyperparathyroidism. These patients are sensitive to digitalis. *Nephrocalcinosis* may occur. Muscle weakness, which reduces the requirement for non-depolarizing muscle relaxants, may occur.

Hyperprebetalipoproteinaemia causes *ischaemic heart disease* and *peripheral vascular disease.*

Hypertension may cause *left ventricular failure, ischaemic heart disease* and *cerebrovascular accidents.* Correct dehydration and electrolyte deficiencies preoperatively. Induce anaesthesia slowly, using small doses of any induction agent except ketamine. Intubate gently. Prevent hypotension, hypertension, hypoxia and hypercarbia. Replace fluids accurately as they are lost. Treat hypertension with phentolamine or sodium nitroprusside (see Appendix 3). Treat hypotension with metaraminol. Give large doses of atropine for bradycardia. Postoperatively, rebound hypertension (diastolic pressure greater than 120 mmHg) should be treated with hydrallazine 5–10 mg IV. This may be repeated after 15 minutes.

Hypertension, benign intracranial. See *Intracranial pressure, raised.*

Hyperthyroidism. X-ray the thoracic inlet to show tracheal narrowing which may make intubation difficult. Give a heavy sedative premedication. Avoid atropine. Induce anaesthesia with thiopentone unless the airway is compromised. Intubate with an armoured tube. Ventilate with fentanyl and a non-depolarizing relaxant, giving at least 30% oxygen. Protect the eyes, especially if the patient has exophthalmos. Monitor the patient closely, watching for hypotension secondary to air embolism, hypertension, dysrhythmias and pyrexia. Prevent hypercarbia. Halothane, enflurane and trichloroethylene are contraindicated. In treated patients a thyrotoxic storm is rare. In untreated patients it may occur. Cool the patient with a water blanket and cold intravenous fluids. Give carbimazole 80–100 mg orally if the patient will tolerate it, and sodium iodide 0.5 mg in 2 ml water for injection IV. Treat dysrhythmias with propranolol 1–2 mg IV. Diazepam 5–10 mg IM or IV may be required for sedation. Ensure that hypoxia does not occur. Postoperatively, look for respiratory obstruction due to tracheal collapse or recurrent laryngeal nerve palsy if the goitre has been removed. In untreated patients, close monitoring is required for 72 hours postoperatively as a thyrotoxic storm may occur in this period. Non-depolarizing muscle relaxants may be inadequately antagonized by neostigmine in the presence of thyrotoxic neuropathy.

Hypoparathyroidism. Avoid preoperative sedation. Use decreased doses of induction agents and non-depolarizing muscle relaxants. Postoperative hypocalcaemia may cause stridor and tetany. Treat with 10% calcium chloride 10 ml.

Hypopituitarism. Controlled patients will be taking *steroids* and thyroxine. Give steroid cover. Avoid premedication. Use small doses of induction agents, narcotic analgesics, non-depolarizing muscle relaxants and volatile agents. Replace fluid losses meticulously. Keep the patient warm.

Uncontrolled cases should be given L-tri-iodothyronine 25 μg IV preoperatively, monitoring the ECG for signs of myocardial ischaemia. Cautiously rewarm the patient and give steroid cover. Correct fluid and electrolyte abnormalities. These patients tend to retain sodium and water. Use small doses of anaesthetic agents, and prevent hypoxia and hypotension. Give 5% dextrose solution cautiously to prevent overtransfusion. Monitor the blood sugar, and give 50% dextrose to treat hypoglycaemia.

In spite of these precautions, recovery may be prolonged.

Hypothyroidism. Untreated patients benefit in a few hours from L-tri-iodothyronine 10–20 µg IV. Give also hydrocortisone 100 mg IV. Monitor the ECG for signs of myocardial ischaemia. Correct any electrolyte deficiencies preoperatively. Inject reduced doses of induction agents very slowly. Prevent hypotension, hypoxia and fluid overload. If IPPV is used, reduce the minute volume to prevent hypocarbia. If vasopressors are used to treat hypotension, use reduced doses to prevent ventricular dysrhythmias. Keep the patient warm. Use muscle relaxants, analgesics and volatile agents in reduced doses.

Idiopathic thrombocytopenia. *Steroids* may be used for treatment. A platelet transfusion may be necessary preoperatively.

IgM gammopathy. These patients are prone to *deep vein thrombosis* and pulmonary *embolism* due to increased blood viscosity. Prevent dehydration.

Ileus, paralytic. The problems are similar to those associated with *intestinal obstruction*.

Incontinentia pigmenti. Suxamethonium is contraindicated for tetraplegic patients with active muscle wasting. The disease is associated with *epilepsy*.

Infarction, cerebral. See *Cerebrovascular accident*.

Infarction, mesenteric. Preoperative treatment of shock or replacement of blood and protein losses may be necessary.

Infarction, myocardial. The risks of anaesthesia decrease as the time since the infarction increases, and reach normal levels after about 3 years. In the first few weeks, even a few days' delay will decrease the risk of dysrhythmias. Manage these patients as described for *ischaemic heart disease*. Halothane is contraindicated because bradycardia may allow dangerous escape rhythms to occur. Preoperative beta-blockers may reduce the spread of the infarction but can precipitate congestive cardiac failure.

Infratentorial space-occupying lesion. The patient may be unable to maintain his own airway and have an absent gag reflex. Neck stiffness may occur. Do not forcibly anteflex the neck because this may cause medullary compression. Use a technique which does not cause raised *intracranial pressure*.

Insulinoma. See *Hyperinsulinism*.

Intestinal obstruction. Abdominal distension may splint the diaphragm and cause basal atelectasis and respiratory insufficiency. Dehydration, electrolyte deficiencies and hypoproteinaemia should be corrected preoperatively. The fluid deficit varies between 1.5 and 7 litres. Pass a nasogastric tube as long as possible prior to induction. Aspirate and leave on free drainage. Check whether the surgeon is putting large doses of antibiotics with muscle relaxant properties into the peritoneum. You may object if reversal may be made difficult. Ensure that the patient wakes up quickly and is extubated in the lateral position. Postoperative physiotherapy and oxygen should be given.

Intracranial pressure, raised. The increase may be minimized by utilizing the head-up position, preventing coughing and straining, hyperventilating the patient so that the $PaCO_2$ is 3.5–4.0 kPa, maintaining the PaO_2 at 14 kPa and preventing hypertension. Use adhesive tape to secure the tube, as tying the tube in position may compress the neck veins. For similar reasons, avoid excessive rotation of the head. Giving 20% mannitol 1.5 g/kg will reduce cerebral oedema.

Intussusception. See *Intestinal obstruction.*

Irradiation of the heart may cause *pericarditis* and dysrhythmias.

Irradiation of the intestines causes *vomiting* and *diarrhoea.* Water, protein, electrolyte and blood losses should be corrected preoperatively. *Steroids* may be used to treat the symptoms.

Irradiation of the kidney may cause *hypertension* or *renal failure.*

Irradiation of the larynx. Oedema may last for several months and cause airway obstruction or a difficult intubation.

Irradiation of the lungs causes pulmonary fibrosis. Give adequate oxygen. If IPPV is required, use small volumes at a rapid rate to prevent high inflation pressures.

Irradiation of neural tissue. Active muscle wasting secondary to nerve damage is a contraindication to the use of suxamethonium.

Irradiation of the thyroid may cause *hypothyroidism.*

Irradiation of the whole body causes any of the problems described for specific organs. Aplastic anaemia may occur.

Ischaemic heart disease. Preoperatively, ensure that the patient is not anaemic and has normal electrolytes and acid–base balance. The anaesthetic technique should be designed to provide adequate oxygenation and prevent tachycardia, bradycardia, hypertension, hypotension, hypocarbia, hypercarbia and metabolic acidosis. Replace fluid losses meticulously. Treat hypertension with an infusion of sodium nitroprusside, and hypotension with a dopamine infusion (see Appendix 3). Keep the patient warm to prevent postoperative shivering. Give oxygen postoperatively.

Jaundice. Establish the cause. The prothrombin time is often abnormal. If the patient has been jaundiced after a previous halothane anaesthetic, halothane is contraindicated. Use a halothane-free anaesthetic machine.

Jejunoileal bypass. Preoperatively, check and correct serum electrolytes, acid–base status, renal function and liver function. The patient may also still have the problems of *obesity*.

Jervell–Nielsen syndrome. Myocardial conduction defects may require preoperative treatment with digitalis, propranolol or pacing. Consult a cardiologist.

Juvenile chronic polyarthritis is also known as Still's disease. The management is similar to that for *rheumatoid arthritis*.

Kartagener's syndrome. These patients have decreased immunity (use aseptic techniques) and *bronchiectasis*.

Kearns–Sayer syndrome. These patients have or may develop complete *heart block*.

Kelly–Paterson syndrome. There is an increased risk of regurgitation. Megaloblastic *anaemia* occurs.

Kidneys, polycystic. *Renal failure* develops.

Kinnier Wilson's disease is associated with *hepatic impairment* and *epilepsy*. Avoid giving copper-containing intravenous solutions.

Klippel–Feil syndrome causes *kyphoscoliosis* and rigid cervical vertebrae. Intubation may be difficult.

Klippel–Trenaunay syndrome consists of arteriovenous fistulae which may cause hypoxia, anaemia and thrombocytopenia.

Krabbe's disease. See *Multiple sclerosis*.

Kyphoscoliosis causes respiratory impairment. Ensure adequate oxygenation. Use local anaesthesia if possible. If general anaesthesia is necessary, ventilate the patient with low volumes at a rapid rate to minimize the inflation pressure.

Kyphosis. Treat as described for *kyphoscoliosis*.

Laevocardia. The heart is often structurally abnormal.

Larsen's syndrome. The rib cage is often abnormal. Manage as described for *kyphoscoliosis*. Intubation may be difficult.

Laryngeal foreign body. Give atropine 0.6 mg IM 1 hour preoperatively. Preoxygenate the patient. Then give an inhalational induction and spray the cords with 4% lignocaine. If the foreign body is above the larynx, the surgeon may then be able to remove it. However, if it is impacted and obstructs the airway, a tracheostomy under local anaesthesia may be required. If the foreign body is below the glottis, bronchoscopy will be necessary (see p. 158).

Laryngitis, acute. The infection may spread downwards and cause *pneumonia.* Use local anaesthesia if possible. If the patient has to be intubated, he should be watched carefully postoperatively for laryngeal oedema which may cause respiratory distress.

Laurence–Moon–Biedl syndrome consists of congenital heart disease, *obesity, renal impairment* and *diabetes insipidus.*

Left ventricular failure. Preoperative treatment with a diuretic may be tried. Severe cases should be digitalized, especially if *atrial fibrillation* is present. The patient should be brought to theatre and anaesthesia induced sitting up. During the operation use IPPV.

Leopard syndrome. These patients may have *pulmonary stenosis.*

Leprechaunism. These patients have *renal impairment* and a tendency to hypoglycaemia. Monitor the blood sugar.

Lesch–Nyhan syndrome. These patients may get *nephrocalcinosis.*

Lethal midline granuloma. *Steroids* may be used for treatment. Manage as described for *Wegener's granulomatosis.*

Letterer–Siwe disease. See *Hand–Schüller–Christian disease.*

Leucodystrophy. See *Multiple sclerosis.*

Leukaemia. All types may be treated with *steroids.* Anaemia and platelet deficiency may require preoperative correction. Use aseptic techniques to avoid infection.

Lipodystrophy. These patients may have *hepatic failure, renal failure* and *diabetes mellitus.* Anaemia and platelet deficiency may require correction preoperatively.

Lipogranulomatosis. See *Farber's disease.*

Liver abscess may cause a pleural effusion, which should be drained preoperatively.

Liver failure. See *Hepatic failure.*

Liver impairment. See *Hepatic impairment.*

Lowe's syndrome consists of hypotonia, *osteoporosis* and renal tubular *acidosis.* Hypocalcaemia may require treatment with 10% calcium chloride 10 ml IV slowly preoperatively.

Ludwig's angina causes facial swelling, trismus and oedema of the larynx and epiglottis. Intubation may be difficult or impossible. Tracheostomy is indicated if trismus and laryngeal oedema occur together.

Lung cysts. See *Pulmonary bullae.*

Lymphoedema of the face is associated with chronic laryngeal oedema. Watch for respiratory distress after extubation. Meanwhile, give humidified oxygen.

McArdle's disease. Suxamethonium should be avoided if possible because it causes severe myoglobinuria. The effect of non-depolarizing relaxants is not known. If myoglobinuria occurs, give an infusion of dextran 70, ensure that the patient is well hydrated and, if necessary, give 10% mannitol 250 ml to promote a diuresis. Avoid the prolonged use of a tourniquet, which causes muscular atrophy.

Maffucci's syndrome. Correct the anaemia due to gastrointestinal haemorrhage preoperatively. Move the patient carefully to prevent pathological fractures. Avoid sudden changes in posture because orthostatic hypotension is common. Give myocardial-depressant drugs with caution.

Malabsorption causes hypocalcaemia, anaemia, hypoproteinaemia and abnormal clotting. These abnormalities may require correction preoperatively.

Malignant atrophic papulosis. See *Degos' syndrome.*

Malignant hyperpyrexia. The following agents are safe: all local anaesthetics, thiopentone, pancuronium, fentanyl and pethidine. Nitrous oxide usually is safe but there may be the rare occasion when a patient will react to it. The following agents are dangerous: suxamethonium and all volatile agents. Ideally, dantrolene 10 mg/kg total dose orally should be given as divided doses in the 24 hours preceding operation.

Mallory–Weiss syndrome. Lacerations of the cardio-oesophageal junction may cause severe bleeding. As far as possible, empty the stomach of blood prior to induction. Replace blood loss preoperatively.

Maltworker's lung. See *Alveolitis, allergic.*

Mandibular prognathism. Intubation may be difficult. It has been recommended that an armoured or firm (e.g. Portex, Shiley) nasal tube be used.

Mandibulofacial dysostosis. See *Treacher–Collins syndrome.*

Maple bark disease. See *Alveolitis, allergic.*

Maple syrup urine disease. See *Branched-chain ketonuria.*

Marble bone disease. See *Albers–Schönberg disease.*

Marchiafava–Micheli syndrome. See *Paroxysmal cold haemoglobinuria.*

Marcus Gunn syndrome. These patients require atropine 0.6 mg IV at induction to prevent the oculocardiac reflex occurring when the eyelids are touched. Use pethidine as the analgesic. Fentanyl may cause bradycardia.

Marfan's syndrome is associated with *ischaemic heart disease, congestive cardiac failure,* open-angle *glaucoma,* spontaneous *pneumothorax, kyphoscoliosis* and *aortic regurgitation.* Give antibiotic cover. Avoid hypotension and hypertension. Avoid dislocating joints, particularly the temporomandibular joint.

Maroteaux–Lamy syndrome is associated with *kyphoscoliosis.* Anaemia and platelet deficiencies may require preoperative correction.

Mastocytosis, systemic. *Steroids* may be used for treatment. Use aseptic techniques to prevent infection. Correct clotting and electrolyte abnormalities preoperatively. Intubation may be difficult. Avoid all drugs which cause histamine release. Ketamine and pancuronium are safe, and should be used in combination with volatile agents. Keep the patient normothermic.

Meckel's syndrome is associated with congenital heart disease and *renal failure.* Intubation may be difficult.

Median cleft face syndrome. Intubation may be difficult.

Mediterranean anaemia. See *Thalassaemia.*

Megakaryocytic myelosis. Normal numbers of platelets are present but their function is abnormal. If bleeding is difficult to control, give a platelet transfusion.

Meigs' syndrome is associated with a right-sided pleural effusion and *ascites.* These should be drained preoperatively. Anaemia and electrolyte imbalance may require preoperative correction. The cardiac output may be embarrassed due to mediastinal displacement or a pericardial effusion. Use small doses of induction agents and IPPV for removal of the ovarian tumour. Postoperative oxygen and physiotherapy should be given, as atelectasis is common.

Merzbacher's disease. See *Multiple sclerosis.*

Methaemoglobinaemia, acquired. Treat with methylene blue 1–2 mg/kg IV over 5 minutes. If the cyanosis does not disappear within an hour give another dose of 2 mg/kg. Prilocaine is contraindicated.

Methaemoglobinaemia, congenital. See *Haemoglobin M.*

Migraine. Prevent hypotension and anxiety, which may precipitate an attack.

Mikulicz' syndrome is associated with *leukaemia* and *sarcoidosis.* Atropine and hyoscine are contraindicated. Intubation may be difficult.

Mitral regurgitation is associated with *left ventricular failure, congestive cardiac failure* and *atrial fibrillation.* Antibiotic cover is required. The circulation time is slow. Use a predetermined dose of induction agent and suxamethonium 2 mg/kg. Prevent particularly bradycardia and hypertension. Tachycardia and hypotension should also be prevented but are preferable to bradycardia and hypertension.

Mitral stenosis is associated with *atrial fibrillation* and *congestive cardiac failure.* These patients may be anticoagulated. Antibiotic cover is required. The cardiac output is fixed in mild cases and decreased in severe cases. Avoid myocardial-depressant drugs. Use small doses of induction agents. Prevent tachycardia, hypoxia and metabolic acidosis. Maintain the BP at normal levels.

Möbius' syndrome. Chest infections are common. Give pre- and postoperative physiotherapy. Use local anaesthesia if possible. Intubation may be difficult.

Mongolism. See *Down's syndrome.*

Monoamine oxidase inhibitor therapy in the previous 2 weeks. Use reduced doses of barbiturates, phenothiazines and anticholinergics, as they may be potentiated. The following drugs are contraindicated: adrenaline, amphetamine, antihistamines, beta-blockers, dopamine, ephedrine, fentanyl, metaraminol, methyl-amphetamine and phenoperidine. Pethidine and morphine should be titrated in the ward preoperatively to determine the optimum dose. At 45-minute intervals give pethidine 5, 10, 20 and 40 mg IM or morphine, 0.5, 1, 2 and 4 mg IM. The safe dose is the one prior to the dose which reduces the conscious level or alters the systolic BP by 40 mmHg. If a hypertensive reaction occurs, treat with chlorpromazine 50–100 mg IV, naloxone 0.4 mg IV, hydrocortisone 100 mg IV and, if necessary, phentolamine 5 mg increments IV or a sodium nitroprusside infusion. Treat a hypotensive reaction with hydrocortisone 100 mg and a noradrenaline or methoxamine infusion using one-third of normal doses (see Appendix 3). Treat symptomatically respiratory depression, pulmonary oedema and hyperpyrexia.

Morquio's syndrome is associated with *aortic regurgitation* and *kyphoscoliosis.* Extension of the cervical spine is contraindicated; this, in combination with a prominent maxilla, makes intubation difficult. Use an inhalational induction and use respiratory-depressant drugs with caution.

Moschowitz' disease is associated with *renal failure.* A platelet transfusion may be required preoperatively. *Steroids* may be used for treatment. Hyperthermia may occur.

Motor neuron disease. Recurrent chest infections are common due to aspiration secondary to a bulbar palsy. All muscle relaxants should be avoided; if absolutely necessary, use small doses of tubocurarine. Use respiratory-depressant drugs with extreme caution.

Motor neuron disease, lower. Suxamethonium is contraindicated for at least 1 year after the onset of the disease, longer if muscle wasting is still occurring.

Motor neuron disease, upper. Suxamethonium is contraindicated for 15–180 days after the onset of muscle weakness.

Mucopolysaccharidosis, type I. See *Hurler's syndrome.*

Mucopolysaccharidosis, type II. See *Hunter's syndrome.*

Mucopolysaccharidosis, type III. See *Sanfilippo's syndrome.*

Mucopolysaccharidosis, type IV. See *Morquio's syndrome.*

Mucopolysaccharidosis, type V. See *Scheie's syndrome.*

Mucopolysaccharidosis, type VI. See *Maroteaux–Lamy syndrome.*

Multiple myeloma is associated with *amyloidosis* and *renal failure.* Preoperative blood transfusion may be required to correct anaemia. Treat hypercalcaemia with hydrocortisone 100 mg IV or an infusion of potassium. Use all drugs with caution because protein binding is abnormal. Move the patient carefully to prevent pathological fractures. Use aseptic techniques to prevent infection. Intubation may be difficult due to macroglossia. Ensure adequate hydration and take precautions to prevent *deep vein thrombosis.*

Multiple sclerosis is associated with *epilepsy, kyphoscoliosis* and a tendency to *deep vein thrombosis.* Thiopentone and suxamethonium are contraindicated. Induce with inhalational agents, diazepam or narcotic analgesics. Small doses of non-depolarizing relaxants may be used. Avoid all causes of hypotension as the autonomic nervous system may be involved. The most important part of the anaesthetic is the avoidance of any increase in temperature; increases as small as 1°C may precipitate a relapse.

Muscular atrophy, progressive. Pass a nasogastric tube preoperatively because gastric dilatation is common. Use small doses of thiopentone and avoid all muscle relaxants.

Muscular dystrophy. There are several types. Look for involvement of the myocardium and respiratory system in particular. Preoperatively, correction of dehydration, electrolyte imbalance and hypoproteinaemia may be required. Pass a nasogastric tube.

Use small doses of thiopentone and narcotic analgesics. Use hyoscine in preference to atropine. These patients are prone to hypotension. Halothane should be used cautiously. Avoid muscle relaxants if possible; if not, use very small doses. Design your technique so that the cough reflex returns quickly after the anaesthetic is over. Pre- and postoperative physiotherapy is useful if the lungs are infected.

Mushroom worker's lung. See *Alveolitis, allergic.*

Myasthenia congenita. See *Myasthenic syndrome.*

Myasthenia gravis. *Congestive cardiac failure, hypothyroidism* and electrolyte deficiencies should be treated preoperatively. *Steroids* may be used for treatment. Continue anticholinesterase medication throughout the operation. Premedicate with diazepam if necessary. Induce with a small dose of thiopentone or an inhalational agent. Ventilate with nitrous oxide and halothane or enflurane. Muscle relaxants are often not required. Non-depolarizing muscle relaxants are contraindicated. Suxamethonium may be used but the response is unpredictable. At the end of the operation, give neostigmine 5 mg IV and atropine 1.2 mg IV even if relaxants have not been used. Use local anaesthesia to provide postoperative pain relief if this is possible. If not, give small doses of narcotic analgesics and watch for respiratory depression. If the patient does not breathe at the end of the operation, use IPPV and stop all medication.

Myasthenic syndrome. All muscle relaxants are contraindicated. Use local anaesthesia if possible. If general anaesthesia is essential, induce with a small dose of thiopentone or an inhalational agent. Ventilate with nitrous oxide and halothane or enflurane.

Myeloid metaplasia. *Steroids* may be used for treatment.

Myelomatosis. See *Multiple myeloma.*

Myelosclerosis is associated with *deep vein thrombosis.* The patient is often in poor condition generally.

Myocarditis is associated with severe *congestive cardiac failure,* dysrhythmias and *steroid therapy.* Anaesthesia is extremely hazardous. Use local anaesthesia supplemented with diazepam IV.

Myopathies may be associated with *kyphoscoliosis* and cardiac problems. Pass a nasogastric tube preoperatively because gastric dilatation is common. Suxamethonium and atropine are contraindicated. Use small doses of thiopentone and a non-depolarizing relaxant.

Myositis ossificans. See *Fibrodysplasia ossificans.*

Myotonia atrophica. See *Dystrophia myotonica.*

Myotonia congenita is similar to *dystrophia myotonica* except that all muscle relaxants are contraindicated and the myocardium is not involved.

Myotonic atrophy. Manage as for *Dystrophia myotonica.*

Myotonic dystrophy. See *Dystrophia myotonica.*

Myxoedema. See *Hypothyroidism.*

Nephrocalcinosis. Give enough fluid to maintain the urine output at 125 ml per hour.

Nephrotic syndrome is associated with hypertension and *steroid therapy.* Correct hypoproteinaemia with an infusion of human plasma protein fraction or albumin. Electrolyte deficiencies also should be corrected.

Neuroblastoma may be associated with hypertension and dysrhythmias. Manage using the method described for *phaeochromocytoma.*

Neurofibromatosis is associated with *kyphoscoliosis* and *phaeochromocytoma.* Tumours may cause *glaucoma, hypopituitarism, paraplegia, quadriplegia* and *renal failure.* Always anaesthetize the patient as if a *phaeochromocytoma* is present. These patients respond unpredictably to suxamethonium and are sensitive to non-depolarizing relaxants.

Neuropathy, autonomic. These patients are prone to hypotension. Avoid myocardial-depressant drugs, rapid changes in posture and hypovolaemia. Use gentle IPPV so that the mean intrathoracic pressure is as low as possible.

Neuropathy, peripheral, is often associated with an autonomic *neuropathy.* If active muscle wasting is occurring, suxamethonium is contraindicated.

Neutropenia. Use aseptic techniques to prevent infection.

Niemann–Pick disease. These patients may have *restrictive lung disease* and thrombocytopenia.

Noack's syndrome is associated with *obesity* and intubation problems.

Nodular non-suppurative panniculitis. See *Weber–Christian disease.*

Noonan's syndrome may be associated with congenital heart disease and *renal failure.*

Normal pressure hydrocephalus. Prevent raised *intracranial pressure.*

Obesity is associated with *hypertension, ischaemic heart disease*, respiratory insufficiency, hiatus *hernia, cerebrovascular accidents* and *deep vein thrombosis*. Veins may be difficult to find and intubation difficult. Preoperatively, check the blood gases. Many patients are hypoxic. Increased doses of all drugs and inhalational agents are required but less than expected if the dose is calculated on the patient's weight. Use IPPV for all but the shortest procedures. Give at least 40% oxygen. Avoid using inhalational agents, as recovery is likely to be prolonged. Be prepared for greater blood loss than normal. Postoperatively, give humidified oxygen for at least 48 hours. The semi-recumbent position and physiotherapy will improve respiratory function. Local anaesthesia is technically difficult and unpredictable if given via the epidural or spinal routes.

Oculoauriculovertebral dysplasia. Intubation may be difficult.

Oculoauriculovertebral syndrome. See *Goldenhar's syndrome*.

Oculocerebrorenal syndrome. See *Lowe's syndrome*.

Oculomandibulodyscephaly. Intubation may be difficult.

Oesophagus, perforation of. Treat a pleural effusion, pneumothorax or mediastinal emphysema preoperatively. Septic shock may occur and should also be treated preoperatively.

Old age. Elderly patients require decreased doses of all drugs, and are prone to *ischaemic heart disease, hypertension, cerebrovascular accidents* and hypothermia. The skin is fragile. Pressure sores occur quickly. Veins may be difficult to cannulate. Atropine and hyoscine may cause delayed recovery.

Ollier's disease. Move the patient carefully to prevent pathological fractures.

Oppenheim's disease. See *Torsion dystonia*.

Orodigitofacial dysostosis. Intubation may be difficult.

Oro-facial-digital syndrome is associated with polycystic *kidneys*. Intubation may be difficult.

Osler–Rendu–Weber syndrome. See *Hereditary haemorrhagic telangiectasis*.

Osteitis deformans. See *Paget's disease*.

Osteoarthritis. Osteophytes may make spinal and epidural anaesthesia technically difficult.

Osteogenesis imperfecta is associated with *kyphoscoliosis*. Move the patient carefully to prevent pathological fractures.

Osteomalacia. Treat hypocalcaemia with 10% calcium chloride 10 ml preoperatively. Move the patient carefully to prevent pathological fractures.

Osteopathia hyperostotica sclerotisans multiplex infantalia. See *Engelmann's disease.*

Osteopetrosis. See *Albers–Schönberg disease.*

Osteoporosis. Move the patient carefully to prevent pathological fractures.

Pacemaker, cardiac. *Ischaemic heart disease* and *congestive cardiac failure* are associated problems. Check that the pacemaker is functioning preoperatively. Correct electrolyte deficiencies. Induce anaesthesia with a small dose of methohexitone. Intubate having given a small dose of suxamethonium. Ventilate with alcuronium and fentanyl or low concentrations of halothane or enflurane. Prevent hypoxia, hypocarbia, hypercarbia, metabolic acidosis and hypotension. Replace fluids meticulously. Avoid using the diathermy if possible; if the diathermy is essential, the manufacturer should be consulted. In a dire emergency, place the diathermy plate as far away from the pacemaker lead and box as possible. Tell the surgeon to use the diathermy in short bursts. If pacing fails, insert a temporary wire and use a temporary pacing box. While this is being done, give an isoprenaline infusion (see Appendix 3). Treat ventricular fibrillation in the normal way but do not put the paddles directly over the pacemaker box. Monitor the patient's cardiovascular status closely at all times.

Paget's disease. Kyphosis (see *Kyphoscoliosis*), *paraplegia, steroid therapy* and *congestive cardiac failure* are associated.

Pancreatic pseudocyst may cause *vomiting,* obstructive *jaundice* and a *pleural effusion.* Correct electrolyte, water and clotting deficiencies and drain the pleural effusion. Postoperative oxygen and physiotherapy should be given.

Pancreatitis, acute, causes respiratory insufficiency, shock and hypocalcaemia, which should be treated preoperatively. Mortality after surgery is always high. No particular anaesthetic technique has been shown to influence the outcome of these cases.

Pancreatitis, chronic, is associated with *diabetes mellitus* and alcohol and morphine *addiction.*

Pancytopenia. See *Anaemia, aplastic.*

Paramyotonia congenita. Suxamethonium is contraindicated. Keep the patient warm, as cold and shivering may precipitate myotonia. If myotonia occurs, try the same treatment as described for *dystrophia myotonica.*

Paraplegia. Suxamethonium is contraindicated for 18 months after the onset of paraplegia. If the lesion is above T7, beware of autonomic hyperreflexia caused by visceral stimulation. *Hypertension* should be treated with a trimetaphan infusion. Dysrhythmias should be treated but may revert as the BP is lowered. Spinal anaesthesia may block this reflex but may cause severe hypotension. The level of anaesthesia is unpredictable.

In the first 3 weeks after the injury, spinal shock occurs. This includes loss of sweating (keep the patient warm), paralytic ileus (correct water and electrolyte abnormalities), anaemia and hypoproteinaemia (correct if necessary) and postural hypotension (avoid myocardial-depressant drugs, vasodilators, rapid changes in posture and hypovolaemia). Atelectasis is common. Pre- and postoperative physiotherapy may help. Take particular care to protect the pressure areas.

Parkinson's syndrome. Anaesthetic problems occur secondary to levodopa (see Appendix 1).

Paroxysmal cold haemoglobinuria. Keep the patient warm and maintain a good urine output.

Paroxysmal nocturnal haemoglobinuria is associated with *deep vein thrombosis* and *steroid therapy*. Use washed red cells for transfusion.

Pectus excavatum may cause respiratory insufficiency and an innocent systolic murmur. Use IPPV and physiotherapy if respiratory function is severely limited.

Pellagra may be associated with intubation problems.

Pemphigoid is associated with *steroid therapy*, and oral scarring which may make intubation difficult. Manage as described for *epidermolysis bullosa*.

Pemphigus is a distinct disease but should be managed as described for *pemphigoid*. Fluid, electrolyte and protein loss should be corrected preoperatively.

Pendred's syndrome. Manage as described for *cretinism*.

Peptic ulcer, haemorrhage from. Pass a nasogastric tube and attempt to empty blood from the stomach. It may be impossible to completely correct hypovolaemia preoperatively. Use extremely small doses of induction agents and gentle IPPV to minimize hypotension.

Peptic ulcer, perforation, often causes severe shock, which should be corrected preoperatively.

Pericarditis, acute, is associated with *steroid therapy*, and a pericardial effusion which should be drained preoperatively under local anaesthesia. Then manage as described for constrictive *pericarditis*.

Pericarditis, constrictive. Avoid myocardial-depressant drugs, bradycardia, hypotension, hypovolaemia and hypoxia. Monitor the ECG because these patients are prone to atrial dysrhythmias.

Peripheral vascular disease is associated with *ischaemic heart disease, hypertension, cerebrovascular accidents* and chronic *bronchitis*. Note particularly that the action of non-depolarizing relaxants may be reduced at the periphery. Supplementary relaxation may be achieved with small concentrations of halothane or enflurane.

Peritonitis may be associated with shock, which should be corrected preoperatively. Atelectasis should be treated with postoperative physiotherapy.

Persistent ductus arteriosus. Give antibiotic cover. Prevent vaso-constriction, vasodilatation and changes in heart rate.

Phaeochromocytoma, if diagnosed preoperatively, requires at least 3 days for adequate preparation. It may be diagnosed at operation if unexpectedly large swings in blood pressure occur. Stop the operation. Insert two large intravenous cannulae, a radial arterial cannula and a central venous cannula. If the tumour is to be removed, cross-match 6 units of blood if this has not already been done. Allow the surgeon to proceed. Control hypertension with phentolamine 5 mg increments IV or a sodium nitroprusside infusion (see Appendix 3). Enflurane may also be used provided the patient is being hyperventilated. Treat tachy-cardia and dysrhythmias with propranolol 1–5 mg IV or ligno-caine 100 mg IV. After removal of the tumour, treat hypotension with blood. Very rarely, a noradrenaline infusion is required (see Appendix 3).

Pharyngeal pouch. Aspiration may cause preoperative chest infection, which should be treated with physiotherapy and antibiotics if the sensitivity of the organism is known.

Phenylketonuria is associated with *epilepsy*. The skin is sensi-tive. Use Micropore or similar adhesive tape. Monitor the blood sugar, and give a 10% dextrose infusion if hypoglycaemia occurs. Use reduced doses of narcotic analgesics and other respiratory-depressant drugs.

Pickwickian syndrome. Hypoventilation is associated with *obes-ity*. Use IPPV and volatile agents. Give small doses of drugs which may cause respiratory depression. Use oxygen cautiously postoperatively, as it may depress the patient's respiratory drive.

Pierre Robin syndrome. Intubation may be difficult.

Plasma cholinesterase abnormalities. Suxamethonium is relatively contraindicated because prolonged apnoea may occur; treat with IPPV. Fresh blood or commercial cholinesterase may be given.

Pleural effusion should be drained preoperatively unless it is very small.

Pleural fibrosis. See *Restrictive lung disease*.

Pleural neoplasm. See *Restrictive lung disease*.

Pleurisy. See *Restrictive lung disease*. Provide good analgesia so that coughing is not painful.

Plummer–Vinson syndrome. See *Kelly–Patterson syndrome*.

Pneumoconiosis is associated with *tuberculosis, pneumothorax* and *steroid therapy*. Preoperative physiotherapy and bronchodilators may reduce lower airway obstruction. Use IPPV with a slow rate, allowing adequate time for expiration. Increased inflation pressures may be required. Postoperatively, give oxygen but remember that these patients may rely on hypoxia to stimulate respiration.

Pneumonia. Give physiotherapy pre- and postoperatively. Use IPPV and ensure good oxygenation. Postoperative ventilation may be required. Local anaesthesia is preferable.

Pneumothorax should be drained preoperatively (see p. 110). Check that the chest drain is swinging freely before nitrous oxide is given.

Poliomyelitis. Acute cases may have respiratory insufficiency and a tendency to hypotension. Give preoperative physiotherapy. Suxamethonium is contraindicated. Give minimal doses of antisialogogues and respiratory-depressant drugs. Use IPPV during the operation and postoperatively if necessary. Assume that respiratory insufficiency is present in patients who have recovered from poliomyelitis even if lung function appears normal. Use IPPV and low doses of respiratory-depressant drugs.

Polyarteritis nodosa may affect all organs, including the adrenal gland. *Steroid* cover is required. Monitor the patient closely after extubation because pharyngeal oedema may obstruct the airway.

Polycystic disease. Cysts may occur in the kidneys causing *renal failure*, lungs (see *pulmonary bullae*) and pancreas causing *diabetes mellitus*. The liver may be affected late in the disease.

Polycythaemia, primary. These patients have a slow circulation time. Use predetermined doses of induction agents. Increased blood viscosity predisposes to *deep vein thrombosis.* Consider preoperative venesection and replacement with dextran 70. Prevent cold, venous stasis, hypotension and hypertension.

Polycythaemia, secondary, occurs in response to hypoxia. Treat the primary disease and manage as described for primary *polycythaemia.*

Polycythaemia vera. See *Polycythaemia, primary.*

Polymyalgia rheumatica is associated with *steroid therapy.*

Polymyositis is associated with *scleroderma* and respiratory insufficiency and infection. *Steroids* are used for treatment. These patients are sensitive to all muscle relaxants, which should be used in reduced doses.

Polyneuropathy. See *Motor neuron disease, lower* and *Motor neuron disease, upper.*

Pompe's disease. The heart and skeletal muscle are involved. Manage like *muscular dystrophy.*

Porphyria. Local anaesthesia is relatively contraindicated, as it may be blamed for an exacerbation. These patients may have respiratory insufficiency and a labile blood pressure. Correct dehydration preoperatively. There is some doubt about which drugs may be used safely. Choose an anaesthetic technique using any of the following drugs, which are definitely safe: atropine, chloral hydrate, chlorpromazine, morphine, neostigmine, pethidine, promazine, promethazine, propanidid (normal induction dose is 4–9 mg/kg), suxamethonium and tubocurarine. Starvation may precipitate an attack. Give an infusion of 5% dextrose pre- and peroperatively.

Prader–Willi syndrome is associated with *obesity*, dental caries and respiratory insufficiency. Use an inhalational induction and IPPV. Monitor the blood sugar because hypoglycaemia may occur. Pre- and postoperative physiotherapy should be given.

Pregnancy. Throughout pregnancy use the technique described for caesarian section (see p. 158). If the baby is not to be delivered, narcotic analgesics may be given freely. Prevent hypoxia, hypotension and uterine relaxation.

Progeria is associated with difficult intubation and premature *old age.*

Progressive systemic sclerosis. See *Scleroderma.*

Prolonged Q–T interval syndrome. Consult a cardiologist preoperatively because these patients may require betablockers and pacing. For anaesthesia use alcuronium, diazepam, halothane, morphine, nitrous oxide and thiopentone. Atropine, lignocaine, pancuronium, phenothiazines and procainamide are contraindicated. Prepare the defibrillator because sudden ventricular fibrillation may occur.

Prosthetic heart valves. All patients should be given antibiotic cover. Some may be taking anticoagulants, which should be continued unless life-threatening haemorrhage occurs.

Pseudocholinesterase deficiency. See *Plasma cholinesterase abnormalities.*

Pseudohypoparathyroidism. See *Albright's osteodystrophy.*

Pseudoxanthoma elasticum. See *Groenblad–Strandberg syndrome.*

Psoriasis is associated with *steroid therapy* and difficult intubation due to cricoarytenoid arthritis.

Pulmonary alveolar proteinosis. High concentrations of oxygen may be required. Bronchial lavage may improve the oxygen-diffusing capacity.

Pulmonary bullae may increase in size if nitrous oxide is given. Rupture may cause a tension pneumothorax. Use local anaesthesia if possible. If IPPV is used, allow adequate time for expiration, and if necessary increase the minute volume to overcome the leak. Consider the use of a Robertshaw tube if the bullae are confined to one lung.

Pulmonary haemorrhage. Treat the patient as described for bronchopleural *fistula.* Isolate the affected lung with a Robertshaw tube. If one is not immediately available, pass a long cuffed endotracheal tube into the bronchus of the good lung. Subsequent technique will depend on how the surgeon intends to treat the haemorrhage.

Pulmonary stenosis is associated with *right ventricular failure* and *carcinoid syndrome.* Give antibiotic cover. Prevent hypoxia and hypotension.

Pulseless disease. See *Aortic arch syndrome.*

Pyelonephritis, acute. Treat dehydration and pyrexia preoperatively.

Pyelonephritis, chronic. Treat dehydration and electrolyte deficiencies preoperatively.

Pyloric stenosis. Treat dehydration and electrolyte deficiencies preoperatively. Pass a nasogastric or stomach tube and remove stomach contents before induction.

Quadriplegia. IPPV is required if the lesion is above C3. Anaesthetic problems are similar to those described for *paraplegia.* Pre- and postoperative physiotherapy should be given because chest infections are common.

Quinsy. See *Tonsillar abscess.*

Raynaud's disease. The anaesthetic technique depends on associated diseases such as *scleroderma, systemic lupus erythematosus, rheumatoid arthritis* and *phaeochromocytoma.* The core/skin temperature difference is greater than normal.

Recurrent laryngeal nerve palsy of long standing may cause cricoarytenoid arthritis and, hence, intubation difficulties.

Red cell aplasia. See *Blackfan–Diamond syndrome.*

Refsum's disease is associated with respiratory insufficiency. Pre- and postoperative physiotherapy may be required. Use local anaesthesia if possible. Suxamethonium is contraindicated if muscle wasting is occurring.

Reiter's disease is associated with *steroid therapy* and intubation difficulties.

Renal failure is associated with anaemia which is well tolerated and should not be corrected, hyperkalaemia and metabolic acidosis which should be corrected preoperatively, *hepatitis B* and *hypertension.* Gallamine, methoxyflurane and enflurane are contraindicated. Aseptic techniques should be employed. Use a small dose of thiopentone or methohexitone for induction. Suxamethonium should only be used if the serum potassium is normal. Provide muscle relaxation with one-third to one-half normal doses of tubocurarine or pancuronium. Maintain anaesthesia with nitrous oxide, fentanyl and low concentrations of halothane. Prevent hypoxia and hypotension. Replace blood loss if necessary and give an intravenous infusion of dextrose saline solution so that the patient receives 10 ml/kg per day. Severe hypertension should be treated with a sodium nitroprusside infusion (see Appendix 3). Treat hypotension with a dopamine infusion if the fluid balance is correct. Reverse with normal doses of neostigmine and atropine. Give oxygen postoperatively.

NB. Veins and arteries are precious to patients with renal failure. Avoid damaging them unnecessarily. Protect arteriovenous fistulae. Do not use them for injections or intravenous infusions. Avoid prolonged pressure (e.g. from the blood pressure cuff) which may cause the fistula to clot.

Renal impairment. Use reduced doses of drugs. If in doubt, manage as described for *renal failure.*

Restrictive lung disease. Local anaesthesia should be used if possible; if not, use IPPV to reduce the work of breathing. High inflation pressures may be required. Ensure that oxygenation is adequate. Consider postoperative ventilation if the patient is very poorly; weaning is usually easy.

Rheumatic fever is associated with *pericarditis* and *steroid therapy*. Drain a pericardial effusion under local anaesthesia. Avoid general anaesthesia if possible.

Rheumatoid arthritis is associated with *ischaemic heart disease, congestive cardiac failure, restrictive lung disease, pleural effusion, amyloidosis, steroid therapy, osteoporosis* and bleeding problems secondary to treatment. Do not hyperextend the neck; this adds to other problems which may make intubation extremely difficult. The skin is fragile. Prevent shearing and pressure sores. Contractures may make positioning of the patient difficult. There may be the added problem of *old age*. Use local anaesthesia if possible. Spinal and epidural anaesthesia may be technically impossible.

Rickets is associated with *kyphoscoliosis* and intubation difficulties. Treat hypocalcaemia with 10% calcium chloride 10 ml slowly IV. Spinal and epidural anaesthesia may be technically difficult.

Rieger's syndrome may be associated with *dystrophia myotonica* or *myopathies*. Intubation may be difficult.

Right ventricular failure. Preoperative treatment is directed towards improving the causative disease. This is often impossible. Digitalis may help, especially if *left ventricular failure* is present.

Riley–Day syndrome. See *Dysautonomia, familial*.

Romano–Ward syndrome. See *Prolonged Q–T interval syndrome*.

Romberg's syndrome. Intubation may be difficult.

Rubinstein–Tabyi syndrome is associated with congenital heart disease and recurrent chest infections.

Saint Vitus dance. See *Sydenham's chorea*.

Sanfilippo's syndrome. Anaesthetic problems have not been reported.

Sarcoidosis is associated with *restrictive lung disease*, cardiac abnormalities and *steroid therapy*. Severe involvement of the organs may not cause symptoms. Intubation may be difficult due to laryngeal stenosis. Monitor the ECG because dysrhythmias are common.

Schanz' disease. See *Multiple sclerosis*.

Schaumann's fever. See *Sarcoidosis*.

Scheie's syndrome may be associated with *aortic regurgitation*.

Schilder's disease. See *Multiple sclerosis*.

Scleroderma is associated with *congestive cardiac failure, restrictive lung disease, steroid therapy, renal failure* and *malabsorption.* Avoid skin damage and pressure sores. The veins may be poor. Intubation may be difficult because of oral scarring. These patients are prone to hypotension because their circulating blood volume is decreased. Local anaesthetic action may be prolonged.

Scleroedema adultorum of Buschke. The anaesthetic problems are similar to those described for *scleroderma* but less severe.

Scurvy. These patients have loose teeth. Increased capillary fragility causes bleeding. Vitamin C 250 mg orally in divided doses over 24 hours will improve this problem. Hypokalaemia should be treated preoperatively.

Serum cholinesterase deficiency. See *Plasma cholinesterase abnormalities.*

Sheehan's syndrome. *Hypopituitarism* occurs secondary to postpartum haemorrhage.

Shy–Drager syndrome consists of orthostatic hypotension and anhidrosis. Use small doses of thiopentone and fentanyl with suxamethonium and pancuronium for anaesthesia. Maintain meticulous fluid balance. Prevent hypotension by using elastic stockings, employing the lowest mean intrathoracic pressure for IPPV, avoiding myocardial-depressant drugs and sudden changes in posture. If hypotension occurs, give fluid or a small dose of phenylephrine.

Sick sinus syndrome. Pacing is required preoperatively. Avoid halothane and hypoxia during the operation.

Sickle cell disease. Preoperatively, transfuse warm, fresh (less than 5 days old) blood to raise the haemoglobin to 7 g/dl. Correct dehydration, electrolyte and acid–base abnormalities. During anaesthesia prevent hypoxia, dehydration, hypovolaemia, hypotension and cold. Put the patient on a warming blanket and warm all fluids. Postoperatively, give oxygen and analgesics to prevent vasoconstriction. Prevent respiratory depression. Maintain adequate hydration and treat infection aggressively. Tourniquets are contraindicated. Avoid adrenaline-containing local anaesthetic solutions. *Hepatic impairment* and *renal impairment* occur in severe cases. If a crisis is suspected, give 40% oxygen, heparin 10 000 units IV, 8.4% sodium bicarbonate 50 ml IV if the base deficit is greater than 8 and ensure that the patient is well hydrated.

Sickle cell haemoglobin C disease. Manage as described for *sickle cell disease.*

Sickle cell thalassaemia. Manage as described for *sickle cell disease.*

Sickle cell trait. The risks of a sickle cell crisis are less but these patients should still be managed by the method described for *sickle cell disease.*

Silicosis. Manage as described for *Pneumoconiosis.*

Silo filler's lung. Manage as described for *bronchiolitis fibrosa obliterans.*

Silver syndrome. Intubation may be difficult.

Sinus arrest. These patients require pacing preoperatively.

Sipple's syndrome may be associated with *phaeochromocytoma, Cushing's disease* and *hyperparathyroidism.*

Sjögren's syndrome. Atropine is contraindicated. Intubation may be difficult. Use humidified gases and postoperative oxygen.

Smith–Lemli–Opitz syndrome is associated with recurrent chest infections and difficulty with intubation and airway maintenance.

Sotos' syndrome. Intubation and airway maintenance may be difficult.

Spina bifida. Although the lower motor neurons are damaged, problems have not occurred when suxamethonium is used. Use anaesthetic areas for injections and intravenous infusions.

Steinert's disease. See *Dystrophia myotonica.*

Steroid therapy. Steroid cover is required if the patient has taken steroids in the previous 2 years. This is probably an overestimate of the danger period. Current use of steroids may be associated with problems similar to those seen in *Cushing's disease.*

Stevens–Johnson syndrome may be associated with *steroid therapy, pleural effusion, pneumonia, pneumothorax, myocarditis, pericarditis* and *atrial fibrillation.* Correct fluid and electrolyte deficiencies preoperatively. In spite of possible intubation problems, take care to avoid trauma to the airway. Local anaesthesia should be used if possible. Avoid IPPV if possible. If pulmonary infection is severe, the anaesthetic apparatus may require decontamination postoperatively.

Still's disease. The problems are similar to those described for *rheumatoid arthritis.*

Sturge–Weber syndrome. *Epilepsy* is the major problem.

Subarachnoid haemorrhage may be associated with *hypertension.* Maintain the BP at the preoperative level. Avoid hypertension and hypotension relative to the preoperative level. Maintain good oxygenation.

Subdural haematoma. See *Intracranial pressure, raised.*

Sulphaemoglobinaemia. There is no specific treatment. Maintain good oxygenation.

Superior vena caval obstruction. The action of intravenous induction agents is delayed if injected into an upper limb. The intravenous cannula should be inserted in a foot.

Sydenham's chorea. Fix intravenous cannulae well because involuntary movements may dislodge them. Premedicate with diazepam. Manage anaesthesia as described for *rheumatic fever.*

Syphilis may cause aortitis. See *Aortic arch syndrome* for management.

Syringobulbia. Aspiration leads to recurrent chest infections. Pre- and postoperative physiotherapy may be necessary.

Syringomyelia may be associated with *kyphoscoliosis* and *syringobulbia.* Avoid raising the intracranial pressure because this may be transmitted and damage the spinal cord. Correct dehydration and electrolyte deficiencies preoperatively. Suxamethonium is contraindicated if there has been recent sudden paralysis. Use decreased doses of non-depolarizing muscle relaxants. Monitor the ECG for dysrhythmias, and temperature because thermal regulation is impaired.

Systemic lupus erythematosus may be associated with *steroid therapy, congestive cardiac failure, pleurisy, pleural effusion, restrictive lung disease, hepatic impairment, renal impairment* and *myasthenia gravis.* Anaemia and platelet deficiency may require treatment preoperatively. Blistering of the skin may make the efficient use of a face mask difficult. Try using cotton wool padding. Intubation may be difficult.

Systemic sclerosis. See *Scleroderma.*

Takayasu's disease. See *Aortic arch syndrome.*

Tangier disease. See *Analphalipoproteinaemia.*

Tay–Sachs disease. There are no anaesthetic problems.

Temporal arteritis. See *Cranial arteritis.*

Tetanus. The patient's spasms should already have been controlled with IPPV, tubocurarine and diazepam. Suxamethonium and pancuronium are contraindicated. Toxic *myocarditis* may occur. For anaesthesia, use nitrous oxide and fentanyl. Autonomic crises may occur and should be treated symptomatically with hypotensive and anti-dysrhythmic drugs.

Thalassaemia major is associated with *hepatic failure* and *renal failure.* Death usually supervenes before puberty. Anaemia should be corrected preoperatively. Desferrioxamine 15 mg/kg per hour should be infused with the blood. Intubation may be difficult.

Thalassaemia minor. The management is as described for *thalasaaemia major.*

Third and fourth arch syndrome. See *Di George's syndrome.*

Thomsen's disease. See *Myotonia congenita.*

Thrombasthenia. Try a platelet transfusion to correct uncontrollable bleeding.

Thromboangiitis obliterans. See *Buerger's disease.*

Thrombocytopenic purpura, idiopathic, is associated with *steroid therapy.* Transfuse platelets preoperatively. Use fresh whole blood for life-threatening haemorrhage. Spinal and epidural anaesthesia are contraindicated.

Thrombocytopenic purpura, secondary. The management is as described for idiopathic *thrombocytopenic purpura* (above).

Thrombocytopenic purpura, thrombotic. See *Moschowitz' disease.*

Thyroiditis is associated with *steroid therapy.*

Thyrotoxicosis. See *Hyperthyroidism.*

Tietze's syndrome. Intubation may be difficult.

Tonsillar abscess should be needled prior to induction to reduce its size. Trismus may be present. With the patient in the head-down position, use an inhalational induction. If it is possible to ventilate the patient manually, suxamethonium may be given. Pass a nasal tube down the opposite side or an oral tube and intubate the trachea under direct vision. If the abscess is very large, intubation may be impossible. A tracheostomy should be performed. Use local anaesthesia if possible for concomitant operations.

Torsion dystonia may be associated with *kyphoscoliosis, torticollis* and a rigid cervical spine. Intubation may be difficult.

Torticollis. Use an armoured tube. Intubation is usually easy.

Total lipoatrophy. See *Lipodystrophy.*

Tracheobronchopathica osteochondroplastica. Intubation may be difficult due to bony protuberances in the trachea.

Tracheostomy. Change the tube if necessary to a type which can be connected to a catheter mount. Thiopentone or inhalational agents may be used for induction.

Transient ischaemic attacks. Carotid endarterectomy is the treatment of choice (see p. 159).

Transplant, heart. The transplanted heart is denervated. Prevent hypotension, hypertension and hypoxia. *Steroid* cover will be required.

Transplant, kidney. *Steroid* cover will be required. Enflurane and methoxyflurane are contraindicated. Prevent hypotension and hypoxia. These patients may be hypertensive if their own diseased kidneys have not been removed (see *Hypertension*).

Trauma, chest

Pneumothorax: may be secondary to fractured ribs or a sucking chest wound. A chest drain should be inserted preoperatively (see p. 110). Seal the wound with a dressing.

Haemothorax. A chest drain should be inserted preoperatively in the sixth intercostal space at the mid-axillary line. Give blood preoperatively if necessary.

Lung contusion. Give oxygen pre- and postoperatively. Restrict clear fluids to 50 ml per hour.

Ruptured trachea or bronchus: may cause massive surgical emphysema or inability to reinflate the lung after a chest drain has been inserted. Bronchoscopy may be required to confirm the diagnosis. If a bronchus is ruptured, pass a Robertshaw tube prior to thoracotomy and repair. If the trachea is ruptured, continue the anaesthetic through the bronchoscope until a tracheostomy has been performed. If the rupture is too low for a tracheostomy, it may be necessary for the surgeon to intubate each bronchus individually until the trachea has been repaired. Postoperatively, spontaneous respiration should be encouraged.

Ruptured diaphragm: the bowels migrate into the chest and compress the lung. A Robertshaw tube should be used. Until the lung on the affected side is collapsed, high inflation pressures may be required. Ensure adequate oxygenation at all times.

Cardiac contusion. Treat these patients as if they have had a myocardial *infarction.*

Cardiac tamponade: See *Cardiac tamponade.*

Ruptured aorta. Surgical repair often necessitates cardiopulmonary bypass. Ask a senior colleague for assistance.

Ruptured vena cava. If the superior vena cava is ruptured, put intravenous cannulae in the feet. Use the arms if the inferior vena cava is ruptured.

Ruptured oesophagus: See *Oesophagus, perforation of.*

Trauma, eye. See p. 162 for technique.

Trauma, head, is often associated with a fractured cervical spine (see *Trauma, neck: cervical spine*). Prevent raised *intracranial pressure*. During anaesthesia use only nitrous oxide, volatile agents and muscle relaxants. Remember to hyperventilate the patient before using volatile agents. Postoperatively, avoid sedative drugs. If pain occurs, give codeine phosphate 40–60 mg IM. Nurse the patient with the head raised. Limit crystalloid fluids to 50 ml per hour.

Trauma, liver. Resuscitate the patient preoperatively. It may be necessary to give more blood than is actually lost, as splanchnic sequestration occurs. Anaesthetize the patient in the same way as described for *hepatic failure*. Monitor the blood sugar if part of the liver is resected.

Trauma, maxillofacial, may be associated with a head injury or cervical spine fracture. Pass a nasogastric tube and aspirate blood from the stomach. Use an inhalational induction. The face may need padding to ensure a good fit of the face mask. When the patient is asleep, gently insert a laryngoscope. If the larynx is easily seen, suxamethonium may be given to facilitate intubation. If intubation may be difficult, deepen the anaesthesia and intubate without relaxation. Choose a cuffed nasal or cuffed oral tube, depending on the surgeon's requirements. Protect the upper airway with a throat pack. Do not forget to remove the pack when it is no longer required. Atropine should be given if the maxilla is to be disimpacted, as this manoeuvre may initiate the oculocardiac reflex. Watch the patient closely postoperatively because airway obstruction may occur.

Trauma, neck

Soft tissue injury. The airway should be secured. Pass a tube by the usual route or, if the throat and trachea have been cut, through the wound. Some laryngeal injuries render intubation impossible. A tracheostomy should be performed under local anaesthesia before an attempt is made to repair the damage. Some injuries are associated with a pneumothorax (see *Trauma, chest*). All injuries may be complicated by air embolism.

Cervical spine. During intubation ask the surgeon to hold the patient's head firmly in the position least likely to damage the spinal cord. In particular, avoid flexion and rotation.

Trauma, skeleton. These patients may require preoperative resuscitation. The following list should be used as a guide as to how much blood is required.

Soft tissue swelling (1 patient fist)	0.5 litre
Fractured tibia	0.5–2.0 litres
Fractured femur	0.4–1.7 litres
Fractured pelvis	2–3 litres
Fractured ribs	1.5–2 litres

Use the BP, CVP, peripheral venous filling and urine output as a guide to the adequacy of blood replacement.

Trauma, soft tissue. If muscle damage is extensive, suxamethonium is contraindicated from a few hours after the injury. Lesser degrees of muscle trauma are associated with hyperkalaemia following suxamethonium from 15–90 days after the injury.

Trauma, spinal cord. See *Paraplegia* and *Quadriplegia.*

Trauma, spine (lumbar and thoracic). Move the patient with care, ensuring that the spine is kept rigid in a 'straight' line.

Trauma, spleen. Preoperative resuscitation should be attempted but an increase in blood pressure may aggravate the haemorrhage. If this occurs, immediate surgery is indicated.

Treacher–Collins syndrome. Intubation may be difficult.

Tricuspid regurgitation is usually secondary to other cardiac diseases. Antibiotic cover should be given.

Tricuspid stenosis causes *right ventricular failure* and is often associated with other valve lesions or *carcinoid syndrome.*

Trypanosomiasis (African) may be associated with *pneumonia, pleural effusion, congestive cardiac failure* and *renal failure.*

Trypanosomiasis (American) may be associated with *renal impairment* and *myocarditis.*

Tuberculosis, pulmonary. Tracheal deviation may make intubation difficult. All equipment should be sterilized after use.

Tuberous sclerosis is associated with *epilepsy,* dysrhythmias, *pulmonary bullae* and *renal failure.*

Turner's syndrome may be associated with *pulmonary stenosis, coarctation of the aorta* and *renal impairment.* Intubation may be difficult.

Turner's syndrome, male. See *Noonan's syndrome.*

Ulcerative colitis may be associated with *ankylosing spondylitis, hepatic impairment, deep vein thrombosis* and *steroid therapy.* Correct water, electrolyte and protein deficiencies preoperatively.

Unilateral facial agenesis. Intubation may be difficult.

Uraemic syndrome is associated with *congestive cardiac failure, hypertension, myocarditis, pericarditis* and *pneumonia.* Correct dehydration, electrolyte deficiencies and protein deficiency

preoperatively. The platelets are qualitatively abnormal; therefore, a platelet transfusion should be given preoperatively. Spinal
anaesthesia (after clotting abnormalities have been corrected)
has been suggested for these patients.

Urbach–Wiethe disease. Intubation may be difficult due to
laryngeal or pharyngeal deposits.

Uveoparotid fever. See *Sarcoidosis*.

Varices, oesophageal, is associated with *hepatic impairment* or
failure. Blood loss may be massive. Insert at least two intravenous
cannulae. Do not pass a nasogastric tube. An experienced
physician may be able to control the bleeding with a Sengstaken
tube.

Ventricular extrasystoles should be treated preoperatively with
a lignocaine infusion (2–4 mg per hour) if they are multifocal or
occur close to the T wave, in runs or with increasing frequency.

Ventricular septal defect may cause *congestive cardiac failure*.
Give antibiotic cover. Prevent hypoxia, hypotension and *hypertension*.

Verner–Morrison syndrome. Correct dehydration and electrolyte abnormalities preoperatively. Prevent hypotension because
angiotensin II, which is not widely available, is often the only
successful treatment.

Villous adenoma. Correct dehydration and electrolyte deficiencies preoperatively. Up to 3 litres per day of fluid may be lost.

Viral hepatitis. See *Hepatitis* (B).

Volvulus causes *intestinal obstruction*. If the diagnosis has been
delayed, the bowel may be gangrenous and need resection.

Vomiting. Pass a stomach or nasogastric tube. Vomiting of gastric
contents causes loss of hydrogen ions, sodium, potassium and
water. Bilious vomiting causes loss of bicarbonate ions, sodium,
potassium and water.

von Gierke's disease. These patients are prone to metabolic
acidosis and hypoglycaemia. Give 5% dextrose solution preoperatively and continue this into the postoperative period. Correct
the metabolic acidosis preoperatively. Do not infuse lactate-
containing infusions. Keep the patient warm. Abdominal distension may cause respiratory insufficiency; IPPV should therefore
be used.

von Hippel–Lindau syndrome is associated with raised *intracranial pressure*, polycystic *kidneys*, *diabetes mellitus* and
phaeochromocytoma.

von Recklinghausen's disease. See *Neurofibromatosis*.

von Willebrand's disease. Correct the factor VIII deficiency preoperatively with fresh whole blood or factor VIII concentrate. The capillaries are fragile. Avoid trauma, particularly during intubation.

Waldenström's macroglobulinaemia. See *IgM gammopathy*.

Weber–Christian disease is associated with pericardial fibrosis (manage as for constrictive *pericarditis*), adrenal insufficiency (manage as for *Addison's disease*) and *epilepsy*. Give steroid cover. Avoid trauma, including excessive heat or cold to the subcutaneous fat. Halothane and enflurane are contraindicated.

Wegener's granulomatosis is associated with *pneumonia, steroid therapy* and *renal impairment*. Use local anaesthesia if possible. Intubation and airway maintenance may be difficult.

Wernicke–Korsakoff syndrome is associated with alcohol *addiction*. Thiamine 50 mg IV slowly plus 50 mg IM will produce a rapid improvement. Hypotension may occur during anaesthesia.

WHDA syndrome. See *Verner–Morrison syndrome*.

Williams' syndrome is associated with *aortic stenosis* and *steroid therapy*. Hypercalcaemia should be treated preoperatively.

Wilson's disease is associated with *hepatic failure* and renal tubular *acidosis*.

Wiskott–Aldrich syndrome is associated with *steroid therapy* and recurrent infections. Use aseptic techniques. Platelet deficiency should be treated preoperatively. All blood products given to these patients should be irradiated.

Wolff–Parkinson–White syndrome may be associated with *Ebstein's anomaly*. It may be treated with oxygen, carotid sinus massage, beta-blockers and DC shock. Atropine and gallamine are contraindicated. Give heavy premedication. Monitor the ECG closely at all times, particularly after intubation which may precipitate supraventricular tachycardia. Prevent hypocarbia, hypercarbia and tachycardia.

Wolman's disease may be associated with *congestive cardiac failure*. Anaemia and platelet deficiency may require correction preoperatively.

Wound dehiscence may be due to *scurvy*. Correct dehydration and protein deficiency preoperatively.

Zieve's syndrome is associated with alcohol *addiction*.

Zollinger–Ellison syndrome. The contents of the stomach are extremely acidic. Premedicate with cimetidine and magnesium trisilicate mixture.

Drugs which may interact with anaesthetic agents

The interactions in the following list have not all been reported, but are theoretically possible as judged by interactions known to occur with similar drugs.

Drug	Anaesthetic significance
Acebutolol	May potentiate morphine, hypnotics and non-depolarizing muscle relaxants. Premedicate with atropine 0.02 mg/kg. Reduce doses of drugs which may cause hypotension. Maintain meticulous fluid balance. Treat hypotension with as much fluid as the patient will tolerate and an isoprenaline infusion. Verapamil is contraindicated.
Acetazolamide	Hypokalaemia may potentiate non-depolarizing muscle relaxants.
Acetohexamide	May be inadequate to control hyperglycaemia in severely ill patients.
Allyloestrenol	Increased incidence of thromboembolism. Consider heparin prophylaxis (see p. 25).
Ambenonium	Potentiates suxamethonium and antagonizes non-depolarizing muscle relaxants.
Amikacin	May potentiate non-depolarizing muscle relaxants. Frusemide may increase ototoxicity and nephrotoxicity.
Amiloride	Causes hyperkalaemia which, if untreated, could in turn cause cardiac arrest with suxamethonium.

Drug	Anaesthetic significance

Aminophylline
: Use cautiously with halothane, as both cause dysrhythmias.

Amiodarone
: May cause bradycardia if given with beta-blockers. Treat with isoprenaline. Use halothane cautiously to avoid bradycardia and hypotension.

Amitriptyline
: May cause hypotension and dysrhythmias during anaesthesia. Phenylephrine and methoxamine should be used cautiously for the treatment of hypotension. Adrenaline must not be used. Reduce doses of barbiturates, anticholinergic drugs, pethidine and possibly other narcotics because they may be potentiated. These interactions may occur up to 10 days after the last dose of amitriptyline.

Amphetamine
: Has an unpredictable effect on induction agent action. A recent dose may shorten the duration of action of induction agents.

Amphotericin
: Hypokalaemia may potentiate non-depolarizing relaxants. May also potentiate suxamethonium.

Amylobarbitone
: A recent dose may potentiate the effects of CNS-depressant drugs. Induces liver enzymes, causing increased rate of metabolism of thiopentone and methohexitone.

Ancrod
: Should be reversed if given within 48 hours of major surgery. The manufacturer's recommended regimen is to give ancrod antidote 0.2 ml SC and observe for 30 minutes. If signs of allergy are absent, give 0.8 ml antidote IM and observe for a further 30 minutes. If signs of nodular reaction are absent, give 1.0 ml antidote IV and 5 g human fibrinogen IV.

Drug	Anaesthetic significance
Ancrod, *cont.*	If fibrinogen is not available, give 1 litre fresh plasma or whole blood, watching for signs of fluid overload. In an emergency, give 1.0 ml anti-dote IV with 5 g human fibrinogen, chlorpheniramine 10 mg and hydro-cortisone 100 mg IV.
Aprotinin	May potentiate suxamethonium in the presence of a low plasma cho-linesterase.
Atenolol	*see* Acebutolol.
Azatadine	Potentiates CNS-depressant effects of other drugs, whose dosage should be reduced.
Azathioprine	Potentiates suxamethonium. Antago-nizes tubocurarine.
Baclofen	Causes weakness of respiratory muscles. Use other respiratory de-pressants with care.
Bendrofluazide	Hypokalaemia may potentiate non-depolarizing muscle relaxants.
Benperidol	Use cautiously with other CNS de-pressants.
Benzthiazide	*see* Bendrofluazide.
Benztropine	Reduce the dose of atropine be-cause both cause tachycardia.
Betamethasone	Give steroid cover (see p. 25).
Bethanidine	Causes hypotension with standard doses of induction agents, halothane, enflurane, tubocurarine and spinal anaesthesia. Treat with fluid and metaraminol. Avoid or use reduced doses of direct-acting sympatho-mimetics.
Bleomycin	Never increase the inspired oxygen concentration above 25%. Replace fluids meticulously with colloid rather than crystalloid solutions.
Bretylium	*see* Bethanidine.
Brompheniramine	*see* Azatadine.

Drug	*Anaesthetic significance*
Buclizine	*see* Cyclizine.
Bumetanide	*see* Bendrofluazide.
Buprenorphine	Use decreased doses of other CNS depressants.
Butobarbitone	*see* Amylobarbitone.
Butriptyline	*see* Amitryptyline.
Cannabis	Causes severe hypotension with standard doses of vasopressors. Use vasopressors only if absolutely necessary, and in reduced doses.
Capreomycin	Hypokalaemia may potentiate non-depolarizing muscle relaxants.
Captopril	Hypotension may occur with standard doses of induction agents, halothane, enflurane, tubocurarine and spinal anaesthesia. Treat with fluid.
Carbamazepine	Reduce doses of narcotics because they may be potentiated.
Carbenoxolone	Hypokalaemia may potentiate non-depolarizing muscle relaxants.
Carbidopa	*see* Levodopa.
Carbinoxamine	*see* Azatadine.
Chlordiazepoxide	May potentiate sedative effects of other drugs and non-depolarizing muscle relaxants.
Chlormethiazole	Decrease dose of CNS-depressant drugs, which may be potentiated.
Chlormezanone	*see* Chlormethiazole.
Chlorothiazide	*see* Bendrofluazide.
Chlorpheniramine	*see* Azatadine.
Chlorpromazine	Decrease dose of CNS-depressant drugs. May cause hypotension with anaesthetic agents; treat with fluid, noradrenaline or metaraminol.
Chlorpropamide	*see* Acetohexamide.
Chlorprothixene	*see* Chlorpromazine.
Chlortetracycline	Methoxyflurane is contraindicated.
Chlorthalidone	*see* Bendrofluazide.
Choline theophyllinate	*see* Aminophylline.

Drug	Anaesthetic significance
Cinnarizine	*see* Azatadine.
Clemastine	*see* Azatadine.
Clindamycin	May potentiate non-depolarizing muscle relaxants.
Clobazam	*see* Chlordiazepoxide.
Clomipramine	*see* Amitriptyline.
Clomocycline	*see* Chlortetracycline.
Clonazepam	*see* Chlordiazepoxide.
Clonidine	May cause hypotension with standard doses of thiopentone, halothane, enflurane, tubocurarine and spinal anaesthesia. If a dose has been omitted, give 0.15–0.3 mg IV to prevent rebound hypertension.
Clopamide	*see* Bendrofluazide.
Clopenthixol	*see* Chlorpromazine.
Clorazepate	*see* Chlordiazepoxide.
Clorexolone	*see* Bendrofluazide.
Colchicine	Reduce doses of CNS-depressant drugs, which may be potentiated.
Colistin	May potentiate non-depolarizing muscle relaxants. Try reversing with 10–20 ml 10% calcium gluconate IV.
Cortisone	Give steroid cover (see p. 25).
Cyclizine	May increase abnormal muscle movements caused by methohexitone. A severe anaphylactic reaction has occurred with propanidid. Decrease dose of CNS-depressant drugs, which may be potentiated.
Cyclobarbitone	*see* Amylobarbitone.
Cyclopenthiazide	*see* Bendrofluazide.
Cyclophosphamide	May potentiate suxamethonium.
Cyproheptadine	*see* Azatadine.
Cyproterone	May require steroid cover (see p. 25).
Dantrolene	Reduce doses of CNS-depressant drugs, which may be potentiated.

Drug	*Anaesthetic significance*
Debrisoquine	A MAOI (see Chapter 9). May cause hypotension with thiopentone, halothane, enflurane, tubocurarine and spinal anaesthetics.
Demeclocycline	*see* Chlortetracycline.
Deoxycortone	Requires steroid cover (see p. 25).
Desipramine	*see* Amitriptyline.
Deslanoside	*see* Digoxin.
Desmopressin	Halothane is contraindicated.
Dexamethasone	Requires steroid cover (see p. 25).
Dexamphetamine	*see* Amphetamine.
Dextropropoxyphene	*see* Buprenorphine.
Diamorphine	*see* Buprenorphine.
Diazepam	*see* Chlordiazepoxide.
Dibenzepin	*see* Amitriptyline.
Dichlorphenamide	*see* Acetazolamide.
Dicoumarol	Reverse with 4 units fresh-frozen plasma. If unreversed, avoid IM injections, nasal intubation and regional anaesthesia. Spinal and epidural anaesthetics are absolutely contraindicated.
Digitoxin	*see* Digoxin.
Digoxin	Bradycardia with suxamethonium and halothane may be reversed with atropine. Ventricular ectopics may occur with neostigmine.
Dimenhydrinate	*see* Azatadine.
Dimethindine	*see* Chlorpromazine.
Dimethothiazine	*see* Chlorpromazine.
Diphenhydramine	*see* Azatadine.
Diphenoxylate	Reduce the dose of CNS-depressant drugs, which may be potentiated.
Diphenylhydantoin	May potentiate non-depolarizing muscle relaxants and suxamethonium.
Diphenylpyraline	*see* Azatadine.
Dipipanone	*see* Buprenorphine.
Diprophylline	*see* Aminophylline.
Disopyramide	*see* Amiodarone.

Drug	*Anaesthetic significance*
Distigmine	*see* Ambenonium.
Disulfiram	Decrease dose of thiopentone and methohexitone.
Dothiepin	*see* Amitriptyline.
Doxycycline	*see* Chlortetracycline.
Droperidol	*see* Benperidol.
Ecothiopate	*see* Ambenonium.
Epithiazide	*see* Bendrofluazide.
Etamiphylline	*see* Aminophylline.
Ethacrynic acid	*see* Bendrofluazide.
Fenfluramine	Decrease dose of CNS-depressant drugs. May cause dysrhythmias with halothane.
Fenoterol	May cause dysrhythmias with halothane. With atropine may cause severe tachycardia. Treat with a beta-blocker.
Fludrocortisone	Requires steroid cover (see p. 25)
Flupenthixol	*see* Chlorpromazine.
Fluphenazine	*see* Chlorpromazine.
Flurazepam	*see* Chlordiazepoxide.
Fluspirilene	*see* Benperidol.
Framycetin	*see* Colistin.
Frusemide	*see* Bendrofluazide.
Gentamicin	*see* Colistin.
Glibenclamide	*see* Acetohexamide.
Glibornuride	*see* Acetohexamide.
Gliclazide	*see* Acetohexamide.
Glipizide	*see* Acetohexamide.
Gliquidone	*see* Acetohexamide.
Glyceryl trinitrate	Useful immediately preoperatively to relieve angina but may cause hypotension with standard doses of induction agents.
Glymidine	*see* Acetohexamide.
Guanethidine	May cause hypotension with standard doses of thiopentone, halothane, enflurane, tubocurarine and spinal anaesthetics; treat with fluid, methoxamine or phenylephrine.

Drug	Anaesthetic significance
Guanoclor	*see* Guanethidine.
Guanoxan	*see* Guanethidine.
Haloperidol	*see* Benperidol.
Heparin	If uncontrollable haemorrhage occurs, reverse with protamine 10 mg every 0.5 minute until clot is observed in the wound and on the mops. Spinal and epidural anaesthesia are contraindicated if heparin is unreversed.
Heptabarbitone	*see* Amylobarbitone.
Hexobarbitone	*see* Amylobarbitone.
Hydralazine	*see* Guanethidine.
Hydrochlorothiazide	*see* Bendrofluazide.
Hydrocortisone	Requires steroid cover (see p. 25).
Hydroflumethiazide	*see* Bendrofluazide.
Imipramine	*see* Amitriptyline.
Indapamide	Doses greater than 2.5 mg daily may cause hypokalaemia and potentiation of non-depolarizing muscle relaxants.
Iprindole	*see* Amitriptyline.
Iproniazid	A MAOI (see Chapter 9).
Isocarboxazid	A MAOI (see Chapter 9).
Kanamycin	*see* Colistin.
Ketazolam	*see* Chlordiazepoxide.
Ketotifen	*see* Azatadine.
Labetalol	*see* Acebutolol.
Lanatoside C	*see* Digoxin.
Levodopa	Use halothane with caution to avoid hypotension and dysrhythmias. Droperidol is contraindicated.
Levorphanol	*see* Buprenorphine.
Lincomycin	*see* Colistin.
Lithium	Potentiates suxamethonium and non-depolarizing muscle relaxants. Avoid preoperative dehydration and electrolyte imbalance, which may cause lithium toxicity and prolonged recovery from anaesthesia.

Drug	Anaesthetic significance
Lorazepam	*see* Chlordiazepoxide.
Lormetazepam	*see* Chlordiazepoxide.
LSD-25	Potentiates morphine and suxamethonium. Reduce the dose of thiopentone and tubocurarine to avoid hypotension. A mild MAOI (see Chapter 9).
Lymecycline	*see* Chlortetracycline.
Lypressin	*see* Desmopressin.
Magnesium sulphate	Potentiates suxamethonium and tubocurarine.
Maprotiline	*see* Amitriptyline.
Mebhydrolin	*see* Azatadine.
Mecamylamine	Hypotension may occur with standard doses of thiopentone, halothane, enflurane, tubocurarine and spinal anaesthetics; treat with fluid and metaraminol. Avoid direct-acting sympathomimetics. May potentiate non-depolarizing relaxants.
Meclozine	*see* Azatadine.
Medazepam	*see* Chlordiazepoxide.
Medigoxin	*see* Digoxin.
Mefruside	*see* Bendrofluazide.
Mepyramine	*see* Azatadine.
Mequitazine	*see* Azatadine.
Metformin	*see* Acetohexamide.
Methacycline	*see* Chlortetracycline.
Methadone	*see* Buprenorphine.
Methocarbamol	Use reduced doses of thiopentone and atropine.
Methyclothiazide	*see* Bendrofluazide.
Methyldopa	*see* Guanethidine.
Methylphenobarbitone	*see* Amylobarbitone.
Metoclopramide	Antagonizes the effects of atropine.
Metolazone	*see* Bendrofluazide.
Metoprolol	*see* Acebutolol.
Mianserin	*see* Amitriptyline.
Minocycline	*see* Chlortetracycline.
Minoxidil	*see* Guanethidine.

Drug	*Anaesthetic significance*
Morphine	*see* Buprenorphine.
Mustine	Potentiates non-depolarizing muscle relaxants.
Nadolol	*see* Acebutolol.
Neomycin	*see* Colistin.
Neostigmine	*see* Ambenonium.
Netilmicin	*see* Colistin.
Nicoumalone	*see* Dicoumarol.
Nomifensine	*see* Amitriptyline.
Nortriptyline	*see* Amitriptyline.
Orciprenaline	Atropine is contraindicated because it may cause severe tachycardia; treat with a beta-blocker.
Ouabain	*see* Digoxin.
Oxazepam	*see* Chlordiazepoxide.
Oxprenolol	*see* Acebutolol.
Oxypertine	*see* Chlorpromazine.
Oxytetracycline	*see* Chlortetracycline.
Oxytocin	May potentiate non-depolarizing muscle relaxants.
Papaveretum	*see* Buprenorphine.
Paramethasone	Requires steroid cover (see p. 25).
Pargyline	A MAOI (see Chapter 9).
Pentaerythritol tetranitrate	*see* Glyceryl trinitrate.
Pentazocine	*see* Buprenorphine.
Pentobarbitone	*see* Amylobarbitone.
Pericyazine	*see* Chlorpromazine.
Perphenazine	*see* Chlorpromazine.
Pethidine	*see* Buprenorphine.
Phenazocine	*see* Buprenorphine.
Phenelzine	Potentiates suxamethonium. A MAOI (see Chapter 9).
Phenformin	*see* Acetohexamide.
Phenindamine	*see* Azatadine.
Phenindione	*see* Dicoumarol.
Pheniramine	*see* Azatadine.
Phenobarbitone	*see* Amylobarbitone.
Phentermine	Use reduced doses of other sympathomimetics and avoid halothane.

Drug	*Anaesthetic significance*
Phenytoin	Potentiates non-depolarizing muscle relaxants. Liver failure has occurred with halothane.
Phthalylsulphathiazole	Procaine and benzocaine are relatively contraindicated because the action of the antibiotic is antagonized.
Physostigmine	*see* Ambenonium.
Pill (oral contraceptive)	Increased incidence of thromboembolism. Consider prophylactic heparin (see p. 25).
Pimozide	*see* Benperidol.
Pindolol	*see* Acebutolol.
Polymyxin B	*see* Colistin.
Polythiazide	*see* Bendrofluazide.
Prazosin	*see* Guanethidine.
Prednisolone	Requires steroid cover (see p. 25).
Prednisone	Requires steroid cover (see p. 25).
Prenylamine	Causes hypotension with thiopentone, halothane, enflurane, tubocurarine and spinal anaesthetics; treat with fluid. Avoid adrenaline, noradrenaline and isoprenaline. The use of beta-blockers, procainamide, amiodarone and lignocaine is contraindicated.
Procainamide	May potentiate suxamethonium and non-depolarizing muscle relaxants.
Procarbazine	A MAOI (see Chapter 9).
Prochlorperazine	*see* Chlorpromazine.
Promazine	*see* Chlorpromazine.
Promethazine	*see* Azatadine.
Propranolol	*see* Acebutolol. May potentiate suxamethonium.
Protriptyline	*see* Amitriptyline.
Proxyphylline	*see* Aminophylline.
Pyridostigmine	*see* Ambenonium.
Pyrimethamine	Lorazepam is contraindicated.
Quinalbarbitone	*see* Amylobarbitone.
Quinethazone	*see* Bendrofluazide.

Drug	Anaesthetic significance
Quinidine	May potentiate suxamethonium and non-depolarizing muscle relaxants.
Rauwolfia alkaloids	see Guanethidine.
Reproterol	May cause dysrhythmias with halothane.
Reserpine	see Guanethidine.
Rimiterol	see Reproterol.
Ritodrine	Hypokalaemia may potentiate non-depolarizing muscle relaxants. Avoid atropine because it may cause severe tachycardia; treat with a beta-blocker.
Salbutamol	see Reproterol.
Sodium bicarbonate	Alkalosis may potentiate non-depolarizing muscle relaxants.
Sodium valproate	Reduce the dose of CNS-depressant drugs.
Sotalol	see Acebutolol.
Streptokinase	Reverse preoperatively with tranexamic acid 10 mg/kg IV slowly.
Streptomycin	see Colistin.
Sulfadoxine	see Phthalylsulphathiazole.
Sulfametopyrazine	see Phthalylsulphathiazole.
Sulphadiazine	see Phthalylsulphathiazole.
Sulphadimethoxine	see Phthalylsulphathiazole.
Sulphadimidine	see Phthalylsulphathiazole.
Sulphafurazole	see Phthalylsulphathiazole. May also increase sensitivity to thiopentone.
Sulphaguanidine	see Phthalylsulphathiazole.
Sulphamethizole	see Phthalylsulphathiazole.
Sulphamethoxazole	see Phthalylsulphathiazole.
Sulphamethoxypyridazine	see Phthalylsulphathiazole.
Sulphaphenazole	see Phthalylsulphathiazole.
Sulphapyridine	see Phthalylsulphathiazole.
Sulphasalazine	see Phthalylsulphathiazole.
Sulphathiazine	see Phthalylsulphathiazole.
Temazepam	see Chlordiazepoxide.
Terbutaline	see Reproterol.
Tetracosactrin	Requires steroid cover (see p. 25).
Tetracycline	see Chlortetracycline.

Drug	*Anaesthetic significance*
Theophylline	*see* Aminophylline.
Thiethylperazine	*see* Chlorpromazine.
Thiopropazate	*see* Chlorpromazine.
Thioproperazine	*see* Chlorpromazine.
Thioridazine	*see* Chlorpromazine.
Thiotepa	Potentiates suxamethonium.
Thyroxine	Ketamine is contraindicated.
Timolol	*see* Acebutolol.
Tobramycin	*see* Colistin.
Tolazamide	*see* Acetohexamide.
Tolbutamide	*see* Acetohexamide.
Tranylcypromine	A MAOI (see Chapter 9).
Trazodone	*see* Amitriptyline.
Triamcinolone	Requires steroid cover (see p. 25).
Triamterene	*see* Amiloride.
Triazolam	*see* Chlordiazepoxide.
Trifluoperazine	*see* Chlorpromazine.
Trifluperidol	*see* Benperidol.
Trimeprazine	*see* Azatadine.
Trimipramine	*see* Amitriptyline.
Triprolidine	*see* Azatadine.
Urokinase	*see* Streptokinase.
Vasopressin	*see* Desmopressin.
Verapamil	Use halothane with caution to avoid hypotension and bradycardia. Beta-blockers should not be given within 8 hours of the last dose of verapamil.
Veratrum viride alkaloids	Hypotension may occur with standard doses of thiopentone, halothane, enflurane, tubocurarine and spinal anaesthetics; reverse with fluid or any vasopressor.
Viloxazine	*see* Amitriptyline.
Warfarin	*see* Dicoumarol.
Xipamide	*see* Bendrofluazide.

Appendix 2

Solutions suitable for cleansing the skin

For disinfection of apparently clean skin

Aqueous solution of povidone-iodine 10% w/v

Alcoholic solution of povidone-iodine 10% w/v
Chlorhexidine gluconate 0.5% in 70% w/w isopropyl alcohol

For disinfection of skin contaminated with dirt or grease

Cetrimide 0.5% w/v solution in 70% alcohol

Appendix 3

Drug infusions

Drug	Usual dose range	Common dilutions	Comments
Anaesthetic agents			
Althesin	10–20 ml per hour	50 ml Althesin added to 450 ml 5% dextrose solution or physiological saline solution giving a 10% solution v/v. Use a 100 ml burette if only small volumes are required	Adjust the rate until the usual signs of inadequate anaesthesia are absent. An analgesic supplement is required for painful operations
Diazepam	Start at 20 mg per hour	Use undiluted in a syringe pump	Use a central vein if one is available
Etomidate (for infusion)	*Loading dose:* 0.1 mg/kg for 10 minutes. *Maintenance dose:* 0.005 –0.01 mg/kg per minute	125 mg etomidate is added to at least 50 ml of physiological saline solution or 5% dextrose. Adjust the total volume to suit the pump being used to administer the infusion	Adjust the rate until the usual signs of inadequate anaesthesia are absent. An analgesic supplement is required for painful operations
Suxamethonium	2–5 mg per minute	500 mg suxamethonium is added to 500 ml 5% dextrose solution or physiological saline solution, giving an 0.1% solution	Adjust the rate so that spontaneous movement does not occur

Vasopressors

Adrenaline	160–400 μg per hour	Add 10 mg adrenaline to 500 ml 5% dextrose solution, giving a concentration of 20 μg/ml	Adjust the dose to produce a satisfactory response. Give the infusion through a central vein
Dobutamine	2.5–10 μg/kg per minute	Dissolve the contents of a 250 mg ampoule in 10 ml water for injection or 5% dextrose. Add the reconstituted dobutamine to 250 ml (1000 μg/ml) or 500 ml (500 μg/ml) 5% dextrose solution or physiological saline solution	The dose should be adjusted to produce a satisfactory response. The overall dose range known to produce a satisfactory response is 0.5–40 μg/kg per minute
Dopamine	5–50 μg/kg per minute	Add 800 mg dopamine to 500 ml dextrose solution, giving a concentration of 1600 μg/ml	Adjust the dose to produce a satisfactory response. At higher doses renal vasoconstriction occurs. Give the infusion through a central vein
Isoprenaline	*For hypotension:* 0.5–10 μg per minute *For complete heart block:* 5–40 μg per minute	Add 1 mg isoprenaline to 500 ml 5% dextrose solution, giving a concentration of 2 μg/ml	Adjust the dose to produce a satisfactory response. Give the infusion through a central vein
Metaraminol	Start at 250 μg per minute	Add 50 mg metaraminol to 500 ml 5% dextrose solution or physiological saline solution giving a concentration of 100 μg/ml	Adjust the dose to produce a satisfactory response. Give the infusion through a central vein

238

Drug infusions (contd.)

Drug	Usual dose range	Common dilutions	Comments
Methoxamine	10–1000 μg per minute	Add 500 mg methoxamine to 500 ml 5% dextrose solution, giving a concentration of 1000 μg/ml	Adjust the dose to produce a satisfactory response. Give the infusion through a central vein
Noradrenaline	1–10 μg per minute	Add 2 mg noradrenaline to 500 ml 5% dextrose solution, giving a concentration of 4 μg/ml	Adjust the rate to give a satisfactory response. Give the infusion through a central vein
Phenylephrine	Start at 20 μg per minute	Add 20 mg phenylephrine to 500 ml 5% dextrose solution, giving a concentration of 40 μg/ml	Adjust the rate to produce a satisfactory response. Give the infusion through a central vein
Hypotensive agents			
Hydralazine	Start at 40 mg per hour	Add 160 mg hydralazine to 500 ml physiological saline solution, giving a concentration of approximately 3 mg/ml	Adjust the rate to produce a satisfactory response
Phentolamine	100–200 μg per minute	Add 50 mg phentolamine to 500 ml 5% dextrose solution or physiological saline solution, giving a concentration of 100 μg/ml	Adjust the rate to produce a satisfactory response

239

Drug	Dose	Preparation	Comments
Sodium nitro-prusside	0.5–8 µg/kg per minute. The maximum safe dose is 800 µg per minute	Add 50 mg sodium nitroprusside to 500 ml 5% dextrose solution, giving a concentration of 100 µg/ml	Adjust the rate to produce a satisfactory response. Use lower doses in patients with liver disease or megaloblastic anaemia
Trimetaphan	Start at 3–4 mg per minute	Add 500 mg trimetaphan to 500 ml 5% dextrose solution or physiological saline solution, giving a concentration of 1 mg/ml	Adjust the dose to produce a satisfactory response. Allow 10 minutes between each change in dose because the effect is delayed
Miscellaneous			
Lignocaine	Start at 4 mg per minute	Add 500 mg lignocaine to 500 ml 5% dextrose, giving a concentration of 1 mg/ml	Reduce the dose slowly until the minimum dose required to suppress the dysrhythmia is established

Appendix 4

Statim doses of vasoactive drugs

Vasopressors

Ephedrine	5–10 mg IV *or* 50–100 mg IM
Metaraminol	2–10 mg SC or IM
Methoxamine	5–10 mg IV slowly *or* 5–20 mg IM
Noradrenaline	100–150 μg IV
Phenylephrine	100–500 μg IV slowly *or* 5 mg SC or IM.

Vasodilators

Hydralazine	20–40 mg IV slowly
Phenoxybenzamine	5 mg IV
Phentolamine	5–10 mg IV.

Further reading

This handbook has been designed to provide essential information for the safe conduct of emergency anaesthesia. A successful anaesthetist not only knows what to do, but also understands why he is doing it. This book only gives information about what to do. The reasons why may be found in the books and journals listed below.

Books

BEESON, P.B. and McDERMOTT, W. (Ed.) (1979) *Textbook of Medicine*, 5th edn. W.B. Saunders: Philadelphia, London, Toronto

CRAWFORD, J.S. (1978) *Principles and Practice of Obstetric Anaesthesia*, 4th edn. Blackwell Scientific: Oxford

ERIKSSON, E. (Ed.) (1979) *Illustrated Handbook of Local Anaesthesia*, 2nd edn. Munsksgaard: Copenhagen; Lloyd-Luke: London

GRAY, T.C., NUNN, J.F. and UTTING, J.E. (Ed.) (1979) *General Anaesthesia*, 4th edn. Butterworths: London

GRIFFIN, J.P. and D'ARCY, A.F. (1979) *A Manual of Adverse Drug Interactions*, 2nd edn. John Wright: Bristol

JENKINS, M.T. (1968) *Common and Uncommon Problems in Anaesthesia*. Blackwell Scientific: Oxford

JOLLY, C. (1979) *Local Analgesia*, 2nd edn. H.K. Lewis: London

KATZ, J. and KADIS, L.B. (1981) *Anaesthesia and Uncommon Diseases*, 2nd edn. W.B. Saunders: Philadelphia, London, Toronto

MACLEOD, J. (Ed.) (1981) *Davidson's Principles and Practice of Medicine*, 13th edn. Churchill Livingstone: Edinburgh and London

RAINS, A.J.H. and RITCHIE, H.D. (Ed.) (1981) *Bailey and Love's Short Practice of Surgery*, 18th edn. H.K. Lewis: London

SMITH, N.T., MILLER, R.D. and CORBASCIO, A.N. (Ed.) (1981) *Drug Interactions in Anesthesia*. Lea & Febiger: Philadelphia

SPELLER, S.R. (1974) *Law of Doctor and Patient*. H.K. Lewis: London

STEVENS, A.J. (Ed.) (1980) *Preparation for Anaesthesia*. Pitman Medical: Tunbridge Wells, Kent

THORNTON, J.A. and LEVY, C.J. (1979) *Topics in Anaesthesia and Intensive Care*. Henry Kimpton: London

241

VICKERS, M.D. (Ed.) (1977) *Medicine for Anaesthetists*. Blackwell Scientific: Oxford

Journals

Acta Anaesthesiologica Scandinavica
Anaesthesia
Anaesthesia and Intensive Care
Anesthesia and Analgesia
Anesthesiology
British Journal of Anaesthesia
British Medical Journal
Canadian Anaesthetists Society Journal
Lancet

Index

Note Chapter 9 comprises, in alphabetical order, conditions and clinical features which have particular implications for anaesthesia. Because there are numerous cross-references, any condition or feature mentioned *only* in those pages is excluded from this Index, and the reader is therefore requested to see also Chapter 9. Similarly, drugs which appear only in Appendix 1 are excluded here.

248   Index

Heart (*cont.*)
  transplants, 217
Heart block, 133–134
  bundle branch, 174
  complete, 7, 131, 133, 189
  first degree, 133, 189
  left bundle, 134
  right bundle, 134
  second degree, 133, 189
Heart failure,
  congestive, 177
  right, 127
  tourniquets and, 97
Heart valves, prosthetic, 25, 210
Heartburn, 5
Heparin, 99
  preoperative, 25
Hepatic failure, 189
  causing decreased conscious
      level, 13
Hepatitis, 190
  history of, 3
Hepatomegaly, 12
Hereditary angioneurotic oedema,
      145, 190
Hess test, 15
Hiatus hernia, 5, 191
Hiccoughs, 136
  in paralysed patient, 116
History taking, 3–6
Hydralazine, 229, 238, 240
Hypercalcaemia, 16, 19
Hypercarbia, 114–115, 118, 143,
      152
  postoperative, 148–149
Hyperglycaemia, 144
Hyperkalaemia, 18
Hyperparathyroidism, 192
  causing raised serum calcium,
      16
Hyperpyrexia, malignant, 109
  causing anaesthetic death, 4
  features, 112–113
  sweating in, 115
  treatment, 112–113
Hypertension, 7, 152, 192

Hypertension (*cont.*)
  causes, 122–123
  drug-induced, 123
  malignant, 151
Hyperthyroidism, 121, 193
Hyperventilation, 135, 148–149
Hypocalcaemia, 16, 119, 150
  preoperative, 19
Hypocapnia, causing failure to
      breathe, 139
Hypocarbia, 140, 150
Hypoglycaemia, 115, 121, 144
  causing convulsions, 150
Hypokalaemia, 18
Hypoparathyroidism, 192
  causing decreased serum
      calcium, 16
Hypophysectomy, 25
Hypopituitarism, 193
  causing decreased conscious
      level, 13
Hypotension, 124–126, 160
  carbon dioxide tension and, 135
  causes, 124
  drug-induced, 153
  from intra-arterial irritant
      solutions, 105
  from transfusion reaction, 117
  in hypoxia, 115
  in nodal rhythm, 132
  in shock, 20
  in vagal stimulation, 116
  local anaesthesia causing, 45
  postoperative, 151, 153
  postural, 5
  preoperative, 8
  spinal anaesthesia and, 58
  tourniquets and, 97
Hypotensive agents, 238–239
Hypothyroidism, 140, 194
Hypoventilation, 114, 135
Hypovolaemia, 114
  causing decreased urine
      volume, 12
  causing hypotension, 124, 153
  causing tachycardia, 7, 120